# ❧ NINE MONTHS IN ❧
## nine months out

Manufactured in the United States of America

Cover by ConnekMedia
Interior Design by Geordie Korper
Edited by Sharyl Volpe
Authors' Photograph by Wen McNally,
© 2011 Wen McNally, www.wenmcnally.com
Cover Photography by Wen McNally © 2008

Published by:
Ironcutter Media
4600 Benedict Drive, Suite 203
Sterling, Virginia 20164

ISBN 978-0-98333147-0-7

I dedicate this book to my wonderful husband and best friend Randy, who supported me throughout my schooling to fulfill my dream as a certified nurse midwife. If not for him, I could have never done it, and be able to share my knowledge with all of the moms and moms to be out there.

*Angel*


To my husband, daughters, and to all the moms who have ever been pregnant, had a baby, or want to have one, this book is for you.

*Corry*


To my awesome husband, my wonderful son, and all my family and friends who have always been there with love and support - Thank you! To all the women who have made or will make this wonderful journey of motherhood this is for you.

*Shelia*


To my mother, my grandmother and all the women in my family, and all the women out there who are already moms or going to be a mom.

*Stacia*

# Acknowledgements

*A gracious thank you to all of the following from Angel:*

Frontier School of Midwifery and Family Nursing, Hyden, Kentucky-for a strong foundation to build on for my career in nurse midwifery;

Case Western Reserve University, Cleveland, Ohio, for my Bachelors and Masters of Science degrees in Nursing;

Bobby "Dr. B" Bowden, D.O., for your support and belief in Womanplace Specialties, LLC , Wadsworth, Ohio and your collaboration services and expertise over the years;

Jeff Morris, M.D., Vice President Medical Affairs, Summa Health System (Wadsworth-Rittman Hospital) who was a strong advocate and supporter of midwifery services and a key factor in introducing Womanplace Specialties, LLC, as the first midwifery practice at Wadsworth Rittman Hospital;

All the former labor and delivery nurses who staffed Wadsworth-Rittman Hospital's Birthing Unit and who were strong advocates of nurse midwifery, especially Stacy Kovacs, R.N., former Head Nurse Manager;

Case University Hospitals of Cleveland, where the seed for my desire to be a nurse midwife was planted many years ago as a labor and delivery nurse.

*Corry wishes to extend deepest heartfelt gratitude to the following:*

The United States Sports Academy for creating the avenue to further my passion.

The United States Marine Corps for providing me my first opportunity to work with pre/postnatal moms (active duty and family members), and to create the "Mom's N Babies Getting Fit" Program.

Gold's Gym for allowing me to be a member of their prestigious Fitness Institute and reach so many more moms nationwide.

All my friends and family who have encouraged me to keep going and never stop dreaming - Your unconditional love and support means the world to me!

My clients – I have learned so much from all of you through the years. Together we have endured pain (lunge day), tears of joy (when new babies are born) and major milestones (losing all the baby weight). Keep shining!

My ACSS Gals --- WE DID IT!!

*Shelia gives thanks and expresses gratitude to the following:*

Campbell University –Thank you! It was here that my love of psychology, my passion to learn about human behavior and cognitive functioning, and my desire to help others all began to take root.

East Carolina University –It was a life changing experience... You helped me develop my clinical skills and gave me the tools to take my passion and integrate it. You empowered me to look at situations through a broad-based approach that takes into account the psychosocial, medical, physical, vocational, cognitive, and emotional health of an individual to help them achieve an optimal level of overall functioning.

My clients – It has been a pleasure being able to work with so many wonderful individuals! We have worked on some of the most emotionally sensitive life situations and hopefully our journey together has been one of healing and growth.

To my friends and family – You have been my rock! Your support and love has meant the world to me...

To my ACSS family – You are AMAZING women! I have been so blessed to be a part of something so special! It's been a long journey of love... but we made it!

*Stacia recognizes and gives thanks to the following:*

To my family, Mom, Grama, Dean, John, Elena & SJ, you are who helped shaped me into being who I am. And to my guys, Nick & Brandon, for putting up with all that I do. Thank you all for instilling a love to learn and the ability to communicate.

To my USANA family, most especially Dr. Ladd McNamara & Dave Delevante – I appreciate the knowledge, skills, support and dedication.

To Gold's Gym of Lake Ridge and Fermin de la Jara at Spinal Concepts for keeping me fit and healthy during my pregnancy and beyond.

To my clients who have allowed me to grow and help them heal. Kim & Connie, thank you for believing in what I do & your healing process.

ACSS Ladies – it's been a long process, but it's finally here! It wouldn't have been possible without all of you.

### *From all of us at ACSS*

We cannot thank Ironcutter Media enough for believing in us, our concept and our mission! This book would not have been possible without any of you! Thank you!

The sections on prenatal and infant massage would not have been possible without the help of Rain Weingarten. Thank you Rain!

# Table of Contents

# About ACSS Transitions

ACSS Transitions is a woman-owned health & wellness company dedicated to sharing and communicating the best information to mothers and mothers to be. Our philosophy is Real Life. Real Health. Real Wellness. Founded in 2008 by Angel Miller, Corry Matthews, Shelia Kirkbride and Stacia Kelly, we are a team of four healthcare professionals and working moms.

Our mission is to provide the best pre- and post-natal knowledge available to help mothers navigate the healthcare world. To that end, we each share knowledge about our core areas of focus including fitness and nutrition, nursing and midwifery, psychology, hypnotherapy and stress management.

ACSS Transitions has published *42 Weeks, 42 Tips to a Whole Health Pregnancy*, and co-published *Nine Months In Nine Months Out*. In addition we offer daily tips and information on our blog, and conduct workshops including Mommy Workouts, Nutritional Guidance, Medical Advice, Stress Management Techniques for Moms and Babies, and Massage. We are based in the Washington, DC metro region. Visit us online at www.acsstransitions.com and look for more health and wellness products from ACSS Transitions in 2011 and beyond.

# Foreword

As a former practicing board certified ob/gyn and current author, I've witnessed many different pre and postnatal reference guides. Some guides approach pregnancy, birth, and life after delivery with humor, while others bog down vital information with confusing or downright scary information for already-reticent new mothers. Other books cover only specific topics such as nutrition or fitness.

The authors of *Nine Months In Nine Months Out* have taken a unique approach to providing information about pregnancy. This comprehensive guide, written by mothers and health-care professionals for mothers, is the first of its kind to address all areas of pregnancy and post-pregnancy from both a medical and first-hand perspective. Each author covers her topic of expertise: medical, nutritional, fitness, depression and stress management. Being in agreement with all aspects covered in this book and how each author covers her area, in my opinion it is undoubtedly the most complete reference guide and resource to the critical nine months of pregnancy and the nine months following birth.

Moms-to-be have a voracious appetite for solid, medically-founded and mom-tested information about pre and post natal health and well-being. Websites such as pregnancy.org reach over 400,000 unique visitors per month, clearly illustrating the desire and need for more information about this beautiful yet stressful time in a mother's life. Now more than ever, women are looking for information covering everything from proper nutrition and what to expect at their healthcare provider's visits to how to decrease or manage stress during pregnancy.

Over the last few decades more and more research has revealed that both positive and negative effects that occur during pregnancy not only affect the health, development, and intelligence of the baby during the first several years of life, but throughout that baby's entire lifetime. Even marginal deficiencies of any one of many nutrients, such as iron, B vitamins, or omega-3 fatty acids (DHA) may negatively affect the learning and memory of the child. Furthermore, if that baby is a girl, the positive or negative influences can affect her children. This means that what a woman does, or doesn't do during pregnancy may have multi-generational consequences.

Between the second and sixth week after conception, the foundation for all the major organ systems are created. The embryo's heart is beating at 4 weeks after fertilization. From the fifth to the ninth week after fertilization the embryo increases in size by a factor of 50. The number of cells increase well into the billions. Initial "generic" embryonic stem cells differentiate into specific cell types, tissues, and organs, with complex cellular functions that display miraculous and dramatic cellular complexities. Obviously, the need to protect the cells from toxic substances and provide adequate cellular nutrients is correspondingly just as critical. Vitamins, minerals, and the essential fatty acids (particularly omega-3 fatty acids such as DHA) are among the most important of these cellular nutrients.

Metabolic demands increase throughout pregnancy and lactation (breast feeding). Several government-sponsored studies have shown that the average non-pregnant American is deficient in many of the essential nutrients required to maintain optimal health. As a result, when the average woman becomes pregnant she is further depleted of nutrients as the baby acts almost as a "parasite," essentially stealing nutrients from its mother. In order to make up for the nutritional deficit that is worsened during pregnancy prenatal vitamins are commonly prescribed. However, it is my observation and belief that a prescription prenatal vitamin is simply not enough; that is it does not provide appropriate doses, ratios, and balance of a myriad of nutrients for optimal health of both the mother and baby during this critical time.

Pregnancy is a time for increased proper nutrition and nutritional supplementation, even more so than when not pregnant. It is also a time to be overprotective of the cells of the developing baby from the many toxic substances and negative effects to which we all may be exposed. Poor nutrition and inadequate supplementation with a full-range of safe and properly-balanced vitamins, minerals, antioxidants, and the essential fatty acids can have serious consequences upon the mother and baby.

Gestational diabetes, pregnancy-induced hypertension, neural tube defects, miscarriages, preterm labor, and still birth are all influenced by adequate nutrients not easily obtainable from diet alone. Recommending proper nutritional supplementation with proven quality supplements, well beyond the average prescription prenatal vitamin, was a significant aspect in my ob/gyn practice to optimize the health of the mother and her baby during pregnancy.

It is my belief that except for folic acid, all prenatal vitamins are woefully inadequate in providing most of the vitamins, minerals, and omega-3 fatty acids required in order to make a true difference in pregnancy and breast-feeding. One tablet simply does not have the capacity to contain the ideal amounts and range of vitamins and minerals required to keep up with the growing demands of pregnancy, nor can it provide the quantities and spectrum of nutrients that research indicates may help in the reduction of many common, but serious pregnancy complications. However, there are safe, full-range nutritional supplements available, and many of my pregnant patients made the wise decision to incorporate them into their daily lives, both during and after pregnancy.

Throughout pregnancy, and particularly during the first trimester, women should undoubtedly avoid all toxic substances. Some are obvious; drugs, alcohol, tobacco; while others may not be so obvious. Although avoiding all caffeine during pregnancy would be ideal, it is definitely wise not to exceed one cup of coffee per day. If possible avoid caffeine altogether while trying to get pregnant and during the first trimester.

There are other substances which are commonly consumed which contain no warning label. Aspartame, a common sweetener in many diet products, is one of those toxic substances that should be avoided by women and men alike, and especially pregnant and breast-feeding women. The cells of the embryo are particularly vulnerable to toxic substances primarily due to the fact that the DNA of all the cells of the embryo are more exposed than at any other time of human development and life. The embryo's cells all start as "stem cells," in which any one of them could develop into any cell type and organ. They develop at a rapid rate, and differentiate into their respective cell type and organ system.

The DNA in the embryo's rapidly dividing cells is particularly vulnerable to damage. Damaged DNA may lead to birth defects or miscarriages. (In adults, damaged DNA and mis-repairs may lead to cancer.) Cell membranes, proteins, and DNA are damaged by free radicals from any number of substances that cause a process called "oxidation." Oxidation is the cause of most chronic diseases, from heart disease and cancer, to diabetes to complications of pregnancy.

Almost all toxic substances, e.g., cigarette smoke, caffeine, certain medications, radiation, pesticides, aspartame, and certain food preservatives, generate free radicals, which damage DNA, as well as proteins, enzymes, and cell membranes. Every human being should do their best to avoid toxic substances in order to avoid excessive oxidation and cellular damage. Oxidation can be stopped or reduced with intake of a full range of antioxidants. This is just one of the many important reasons for taking a high-quality nutritional supplement during pregnancy.

Vitamin E, vitamin C, the B Complex vitamins, beta-carotene, cruciferous extract, quercetin, bioflavonoids, and glutathione, are just a few important antioxidants that protect cells. Minerals, particularly the trace minerals selenium and zinc participate in antioxidant cellular protection as catalysts for powerful antioxidant enzymes (super-oxide-dismutase, and catalase) made by the cells themselves. Such nutrients are naturally found in food, but unfortunately not at the levels that can make significant differences in cases of potentially significant cellular damage. That is why it is so important for all people, let alone a pregnant woman, supplement a healthy diet with quality vitamins, minerals, antioxidants, and omega-3 fatty acids.

Due to our polluted environment; water, air, and food, with additives, preservatives, pesticides, and tens of thousands of man-made chemicals we are constantly exposed to an array of various free radicals and toxic substances. Free radicals and toxic substances permeate the body, and potentially damage any and every organ system, including crossing the placental barrier and affecting the developing baby. You would not let your child sleep in a room full of tobacco smoke, chemical waste, and radiation, so why would you not do everything you could to protect your baby from the point of conception?

Concerned women who are newly pregnant, or women who are contemplating pregnancy, often seek accurate and complete information from books to navigate the complexities of this critical time. Some books concentrate on specific aspects of pregnancy, and others focus on the first year of the child's life. Until now, I have not truly seen a book containing complete information that covers the information women are truly seeking, and from a unique perspective.

As my professional and personal goals are aligned with the book's goal of promoting the highest levels of health and well-being for each and every person, I am delighted to whole-heartedly recommend Nine Months In Nine Months Out to moms-to-be and new mothers alike.

Dr. Ladd McNamara

**About Dr. Ladd McNamara**

Ladd McNamara, M.D., an author, lecturer, and a formerly practicing board certified ob/gyn is dedicated to helping people live healthier, happier lives, and reducing the risk of chronic degenerative disease first and foremost through education and lifestyle changes. He lectures, conducts seminars, authors books and audio CDs all regarding the importance of making healthy lifestyle changes, which include a balanced low-glycemic diet, regular exercise, avoiding toxic substances, and the incorporation of a full spectrum of quality supplements; ...that is, pharmaceutical-grade vitamins, minerals, antioxidants, and essential fatty acids.

Dr. McNamara focuses on the benefits of proper nutritional supplementation, which along with other lifestyle changes include slowing the aging process, increased energy, and most importantly maintaining health and reducing the risk of chronic degenerative diseases that lead to excessive suffering and premature death.

You can find more information about him at: www.laddmcnamara.com.

# 9 Months In

# Introduction

**Congratulations, you are going to be a parent!**

Pregnancy is a time of change. Understanding these changes and knowing how to cope with them will help you enjoy this special time in your life. This book presents a number of topics of interest to not only you, the expecting mother, but also your expecting partner.

Why *Nine Months In Nine Months Out*? When you want to cry and feel ready to tear your hair out, when you don't know where to turn, when you want someone to hold your hand, pick up this book. It's why we wrote it. We wish we'd had these resources when we were pregnant!

This book discusses every aspect of pregnancy. Our goal is to keep you healthy, happy and stress free. All of our stories are personal, real stories, not just textbook answers. Although the information in this book is based upon the latest research available, what sets it apart is that we share what really happens during pregnancy, and not just based upon all the moms we work with in our practices, but as moms ourselves. From the medical to the mental outlook, to the physical and beyond, we created *Nine Months In Nine Months Out* to be the book that guides you through your pregnancy as a trusted friend would.

You may have mixed feelings about pregnancy. You may feel joy and excitement about becoming a parent. You may be wondering if you can meet the financial and emotional responsibilities of starting a family. You may be concerned about how pregnancy and a child will impact your life and your relationship with your partner, including your sexual relationship. Be honest with yourself and talk openly with your partner about your concerns. "Will I be a good parent? Is this the right time in our lives? Can we afford a baby right now?" Expressing your concerns can help you come to terms with your emotions. Partners may also feel unsure of their roles during birth.

It is normal during pregnancy for future parents to focus on issues that did not seem important before. Individually, you may both think about your relationship, your childhood, the relationships with your parents, and your hopes for your future family. Again, discuss this with your loved ones and your partner. Keeping communication open is important, and no fear is too little to discuss!

# Pregnancy Phases

The physical and emotional aspects of your pregnancy can be divided into three phases. You may sometimes hear people refer to these phases as trimesters but this is misleading. The three phases don't have a specific schedule and you will transition from one to the next not on a certain day of a particular week, but gradually over time.

## *Early Pregnancy*

Early in pregnancy, most women feel exhausted, need more sleep, urinate frequently, and have sore, tender breasts. Nausea and vomiting, known as morning sickness, are also common. This can happen at any time of the day or night, not only in the morning. Early pregnancy is a very emotional time for a woman. Sudden changes in mood are common, and you may focus your thoughts inward. Emotions are all over the place! Mixed feelings are common for new dads too. They may be concerned about their partner's health. At the same time, men may feel left out as their partners focus on a changing body and emotions.

---

### Importance of Fathers / Partners

Partners can have a positive effect on their partner's pregnancy. Their presence at your prenatal visits and participating in your care throughout your pregnancy helps build a foundation of support and love.

Research suggests that women with supportive partners have fewer health problems in pregnancy and more positive feelings about their ever-changing bodies. Studies also suggest that labor and birth are easier and shorter for women whose partners take part in the process and who are there for their partners both emotionally and physically through the birthing process.

---

Knowing these changes are a natural part of early pregnancy will help you to support each other and resolve some of your own feelings. This is a good time to get involved in having a healthy pregnancy. You and your partner can adapt your lifestyles to include a balanced diet, an ample amount of sleep and exercise, and to eliminate use of alcohol, tobacco, and other drugs. You should strengthen your own health habits now. Working together for a healthy lifestyle will benefit you, your partner, and your baby.

## *Middle Pregnancy*

For most women, the middle of pregnancy is the most enjoyable part. As your body adjusts to being pregnant, you usually begin to feel better both physically and mentally. Your normal energy level returns, and morning sickness usually resolves at this point. Some women may feel sick throughout their pregnancy, and if it continues, this is something to discuss with your healthcare provider. As your baby grows, your pregnancy becomes more obvious to others. You will soon both be able to feel your baby move and may listen to its heartbeat during visits for prenatal care. Both you and your partner will find this to be an exciting time! Mid pregnancy is the time when most couples take childbirth classes to help them prepare for labor, birth, and breastfeeding. These classes offer a chance to learn and work together and can address many of your questions and concerns. Talk about it, and you may find your fears are also fears your partner is experiencing.

## *Late Pregnancy*

In the later part of pregnancy, you may again feel some discomfort as the baby grows larger and your body prepares for birth. You may have trouble sleeping and performing routine tasks that require moving around. Both you and your partner may be impatient with the pregnancy or excited and fearful about the upcoming birth. Women may fear for the safety of themselves and their baby during childbirth, and partners may be anxious about how they will react during birth. These feelings are normal. Be honest and communicate with each other about your concerns.

# Childbirth Preparation

Childbirth preparation classes include information on the physical process of pregnancy, labor and birth and teaches couples how to use breathing and relaxation techniques to help during labor. They offer another way for your partner to be actively involved with your pregnancy and birth as the primary support person. The support person can also be someone other than the father. The support person's role during labor and birth is emphasized. Teamwork between you and your partner is encouraged during classes, and couples are urged to practice their skills together at home. *The goal of a childbirth class is to make you feel as informed and as comfortable as possible.* Any questions that you have from your classes should be written down and discussed at your prenatal visit.

# Labor and Birth

Your support person's role during your labor and birth process is to provide emotional support and physical comfort to you (helping with relaxation and breathing techniques, massage, and taking care of needs like thirst, etc.) and to help communicate with the hospital staff. Your support person is also there to share in the birth of your child. In most hospitals birth is now viewed as a family event, and your partner will be able to see as much or as little of the birth as you may wish. There may be times at which your partner feels uncomfortable or queasy. This is normal and your partner should try to stay and help you through the birth.

Being there and being part of the child's birth is an important and special time. Most hospitals recognize this and provide personal time right after the birth of your child for the family to get to know each other for the first time. Unexpected situations may arise during labor and birth that require the full attention of the healthcare provider and medical staff. In such a situation, family members other than your support person may be asked to leave the delivery room. Some partners may decide not to attend the birth. There are other ways to support the mother such as keeping other family members company while waiting, preparing the mother's room, and taking an active role in caring for the mother and baby after the birth, even before they leave the hospital.

Finally, having a baby is a family affair. Today, families can be defined in many different ways. It is important to remember that *parenting begins during pregnancy and having loving support is important for you and your newborn.* Fathers/partners are important parents, right from the beginning. The more questions you have answered, the more informed you will be to make the proper choices in your pregnancy.

# In Summary

Within these pages, we cover every aspect of pregnancy:
*   Medical & Psychological Considerations
*   Nutritional Guidelines & Recipes
*   Fitness Plans & Tips
*   Stress Management & Relaxation Strategies
*   Massage Techniques
*   Parenting Skills
*   And more…

We as moms look forward to sharing this journey with you. We wish we had 'us' when we were pregnant!

# General Pregnancy Guidelines

These are some general and extremely important pregnancy guidelines. We will go into specific details in each trimester of your pregnancy throughout this book.

## Prescription Medications

While some medications are considered safe during pregnancy, the effects of other medications on your unborn baby are unknown. Certain medications can be harmful to a developing baby when taken during the first three months of pregnancy (often before a woman even knows she is pregnant).

If you were taking prescription medications before you became pregnant, please ask your healthcare provider about the safety of continuing these medications as soon as you find out that you are pregnant. Do not stop your medication without consulting your healthcare provider.

Your healthcare provider will weigh the risks and benefits to you and the risk to your baby when making his or her recommendation about a particular medication. With some medications, the risk of not taking them may be more serious than the potential risk associated with taking them. If you have concerns before your initial prenatal visit, call your healthcare provider.

For example, if you have a urinary tract infection (UTI), you might be prescribed an antibiotic. If the UTI is not treated, it could cause long-term problems for both you and your baby.

If you are prescribed any new medication, please inform your healthcare provider that you are pregnant and be sure to discuss the risks and benefits of the newly prescribed medication.

# Non-Prescription Medications

Generally, you should not take any over-the-counter (OTC) medication until after twelve weeks gestation unless provided by your healthcare provider.

Prenatal vitamins, now available without a prescription, are safe to take during pregnancy. Ask your healthcare provider about the safety of taking other vitamins, herbal remedies and supplements during pregnancy.

The following medications and home remedies have no known harmful effects during pregnancy when taken according to the package directions.

| Symptom | Safe Medications and Treatments |
|---|---|
| *Cold and Flu* <br> *Sore Throat* <br> *Stuffy Nose* | Tylenol (acetaminophen) - Regular or Extra Strength <br> Warm salt water gargle <br> Saline nasal drops or spray <br><br> *ACSS Tip: Use oxymetazoline (like Afrin or Vicks Sinex) or phenylephrine (like Dristan). If you use a medicated nasal spray, stop after three days. Using it for any longer may cause your stuffy nose to get worse!* |
| *Combination:* <br> *Cough and* <br> *Sore Throat* | Any products in the following families of drugs: Tylenol (e.g., Tylenol Severe Cold and Sinus), Benadryl, Robitussin, Sudafed, Actifed, Triaminic, Chlor-Trimeton, Claritin, Zyrtec, Chloraseptic spray <br> Throat lozenges. <br><br> *ACSS Tip: The only active ingredient found to be effective in over-the-counter cough medicines is "DM" (dextromethorphan), e.g., Robitussin DM. Guaifenesin –watch the amount of alcohol in the cough syrup.* |
| *Other ACSS* <br> *comfort* <br> *measures for* <br> *cold/flu like* <br> *symptoms* <br> *include:* | Salt water (saline) nasal drops or spray; warm, wet compress to your sinus area to help open and drain; set room heat on a lower setting to help keep the air from becoming too dry <br> A vaporizer or humidifier helps keep moisture in the air <br> Sleep on extra pillows to keep your head elevated <br> Be sure to drink lots of fluids, such as 100% fruit juices (in moderation) and water to help keep you well hydrated |
| *Diarrhea* | Unrefined bran, 1-2 teaspoons twice daily <br> Avoid foods containing milk products and caffeine <br> After twelve weeks of pregnancy, for 24 hours only: |

| | |
|---|---|
| | Kaopectate<br>Imodium AD |
| *Constipation* | Metamucil<br>Citrucel<br>Fiberall/Fibercon<br>Colace (100 mg, tablets, by mouth, twice daily until bowel movement)<br>Milk of Magnesia (or Fleet's enema at bedtime if other methods fail) |
| *Rashes* | Hydrocortisone Cream or Ointment (use lowest percent of cortisone sparingly)<br>Caladryl Lotion or Cream<br>Benadryl Cream<br>Oatmeal Bath (Aveeno) |
| *Nausea and Vomiting* | Vitamin B6 100 mg tablet OR<br>Vitamin B6, 25-50 mg, three times daily<br>Sea bands<br><br>*ACSS Tip: Prescription medications are available for severe morning sickness. Talk to your healthcare provider if OTC meds do not help.* |
| *Heartburn* | Maalox Max<br>Mylanta Complete<br>Tums<br>Riopan<br>Titralac<br>Gaviscon<br>Pepcid AC<br>Pepcid Complete<br>Zantac<br>Papaya Tablets (as directed on the bottle)<br>DO NOT take antacids that have aspirin (Alka-Seltzer, Pepto-Bismol) or soda bicarbonate (baking soda). |
| *Headache* | Tylenol (acetaminophen)<br><br>DO NOT take aspirin, Motrin, Advil or Ibuprofen. |

Table 1. Safe Medications.

| **Medications to Avoid During Pregnancy** |
|---|
| Aspirin and aspirin based products |
| Ibuprofen products, such as Advil, Nuprin, Motrin and Motrin IB |
| Naproxen products such as Aleve or Anaprox unless directed to take by your healthcare provider. |

Table 2. Medications to Avoid.

If you want to know about the safety of any other medications not listed here, please contact your healthcare provider and/or the manufacturer to obtain all the information possible.

# Illegal and Recreational Drugs

Illegal drugs aren't good for your health at any time, but they are even worse for your unborn baby's health, since drugs are passed to your baby while you are pregnant. Taking illegal drugs – such as angel dust, cocaine, crack, heroin, LSD, marijuana or speed – increase the chance that your baby is born with addictions or serious health problems, or is born prematurely or underweight at birth. If you have been thinking about quitting drugs, now is the time to do it.

Let your healthcare provider know if you are using illegal drugs or if you have an addiction to any drugs so he or she can minimize the risk to your baby. Remember, your healthcare provider is here to *help* you; expect that they will and listen to their advice and recommendations.

# Vaccination Guidelines

Vaccinations have come under intense scrutiny over the last few years. With every flu season, another media flare up occurs. Regardless of the hype, we want you to know which vaccines should be safe for you and baby. Medical recommendations state the following injections and skin tests have no known harmful effects when given during pregnancy:

- Tetanus injection
- Tetanus toxoid
- TB skin test
- Hepatitis B vaccine
- Influenza vaccine – recommended after twelve weeks of pregnancy, but can be administered in first trimester

*Note:* If you choose not to be vaccinated for these items, be aware, you could be harming yourself, your child or even those around you. However, some vaccines are made for a particular strain of virus and mutate each season, so research, and talk with your healthcare provider to make an informed decision.

# Additional Pregnancy Tests

There are a number of medical tests that will be performed over the course of your pregnancy. Below is a list of the most common ones. Depending upon your medical history other tests may be recommended by your healthcare providers.

## *Parvovirus B19 (Fifth Disease)*

Parvovirus B19 is a virus that commonly infects humans; about 50% of all adults have been infected sometime during childhood or adolescence. Parvovirus B19 infects only humans. There is animal parvovirus, but they do not infect humans. Therefore, a person cannot catch Parvovirus B19 from a dog or a cat.

### *What illnesses does Parvovirus B19 infection cause?*

The most common illness caused by parvovirus B19 infection is "fifth disease," a mild rash illness that occurs most often in children. The ill child typically has a "slapped cheek" rash on the face and a lacy red rash on the trunk and limbs. Occasionally, the rash may itch. The child is usually not very ill, and the rash resolves in 7 – 10 days. Once a child recovers from parvovirus infection, he or she will develop lasting immunity, which means that the child is protected against future infection. An adult who has not previously been infected with parvovirus B19 can be infected and become ill. They may develop a rash, or joint pain, or swelling, or both. The joint symptoms usually resolve in a week or two, but they may last several months.

### Are these illnesses serious?

Fifth disease is usually a mild illness. It resolves without medical treatment among children and adults who are otherwise healthy. Joint pain and swelling in adults usually resolve without long-term disability. During outbreaks of fifth disease, about 20% of adults and children are infected without getting any symptoms at all.

### Is there any way I can keep from being infected with Parvovirus B19 during my pregnancy?

There is no vaccine or medication that prevents parvovirus B19 infection. Frequent hand washing is recommended as a practical and probably effective method to reduce the spread of parvovirus. Excluding persons with fifth disease from work, child care centers, schools, or other settings is not likely to prevent the spread of parvovirus, since ill persons are contagious before they develop the characteristic rash.

### I've recently been exposed to a child with fifth disease. How will this affect my pregnancy?

Usually, there are not serious complications for a pregnant woman or her baby because of exposure to a person with fifth disease. About 50% of women are already immune to parvovirus B19, and these women and their babies are protected from infection and illness. Even if a woman is susceptible and gets infected with parvovirus B19, she usually experiences only a mild illness. Likewise, her unborn baby usually does not have any problems attributable to parvovirus B19 infection.

Sometimes, however, parvovirus B19 infection can cause the unborn baby to have severe anemia and the woman may have a miscarriage. This occurs in less than 5% of all pregnancies for women who are infected with parvovirus B19; it occurs more commonly during the first half of pregnancy. There is no evidence that parvovirus B19 infection causes birth defects or mental retardation.

### *If I've been exposed to someone with fifth disease, what should I do?*

If you are exposed to someone with fifth disease, call your healthcare provider and they will perform a blood test to see if you have become infected with parvovirus B19.

A blood test for parvovirus may show:
1.  You are immune to parvovirus B19 and have no sign of recent infection;
2.  That you are not immune and have not yet been infected;
3.  That you have had a recent infection.

If you are immune, then you have nothing further to be concerned about. If you are not immune and not yet infected, then you should try to avoid further exposure to fifth disease. If you have had a recent infection, your healthcare provider will discuss your plan of care.

There is no universally recommended approach to monitoring a pregnant woman who has a documented parvovirus B19 infection.

## *Chorionic Villi Sampling (CVS)*

This is a diagnostic test done by inserting a needle into the placenta and removing a small piece of placenta tissue (chorionic villi) from the uterus during early pregnancy to screen the baby for genetic defects. This is the earliest diagnostic test offered. This will detect chromosomal abnormalities. There is a 1-2% risk of miscarriage from this procedure. This test is offered between 10 weeks and 13 weeks gestation.

## *Nuchal Translucency*

This is an ultrasound that measures the thickness of the neck of the fetus (nuchal fold) in combination with a blood test from the mother. This gives an estimate of risk of Down syndrome, Trisomy 13 and 18. This test has a 90% detection rate with 5% false positive. This test is done between 11 weeks and 13.6 weeks gestation.

## *Alpha Feto-Protein Plus*

This is a blood test that provides a woman and her healthcare provider with useful information about her pregnancy. It is also sometimes called a Quadruple Screen or Quad Marker Screen. The screening test is performed between 16 and 20 weeks of pregnancy.

Substances in the blood sample are measured to screen for problems in the development of the fetus' brain, spinal cord and other neural tissues of the central nervous system (neural tube). Problems with neural tube development can occur such as spina bifida or anencephaly. Neural tube defects occur in one or two out of every 1,000 births. The quad marker screen can detect approximately 75% of open neural tube defects.

The blood sample is also screened for genetic disorders such as Down syndrome, a chromosomal abnormality mentioned above. Approximately 1 in 720 babies is born with Down syndrome. The quad marker screen can detect approximately 75% of Down syndrome cases in women under age 35 and 85 to 90% of Down syndrome cases in women age 35 years and older.

The blood sample is tested for the presence of the following four substances that are normally found in the baby's blood, brain, spinal fluid and amniotic fluid:

- AFP (Alpha-Fetoprotein): a protein produced by the growing fetus that is present in the baby's blood, the amniotic fluid, and in small amounts in the mother's blood.
- hCG (Human Chorionic Gonadotropin): a hormone produced by the placenta
- Estriol: a hormone produced mostly in the placenta and liver of the fetus
- Inhibin-A: a hormone produced by the placenta

The amount of these four substances found in the mother's blood provides an indication that there is a risk that a baby has an open neural tube defect, Down syndrome, or Trisomy 13 or 18. If your screening test shows a higher-than-average risk of having a baby with a certain defect, further tests will be offered for diagnosis. Most women with abnormal screening tests have normal babies.

### *What happens if the screen results are normal?*

When the test comes back normal it means that you have a 98% chance of having a healthy pregnancy without major complications. However, there are no prenatal tests that can guarantee your baby and pregnancy will be completely healthy or without complications.

### What happens if the screen results are abnormal?

Quad marker screen results that are not in the normal range do not necessarily mean there is a problem in your pregnancy.

The quad marker screen is used for *screening only*, which means it can only assess your risk of having a baby with a certain birth defect (it is not used to diagnose the particular problem that may be present). If the quad marker screen results are not in the normal range, further tests such as ultrasound or amniocentesis may be necessary.

Out of 1,000 pregnant women, approximately 50 will have quad marker screen results that indicate an increased risk for having a baby with an open neural tube defect. Of those 50 women, only one or two will actually have a baby with an open neural tube defect. About 40 women will have quad marker screen results that show an increased risk for having a baby with Down syndrome and one or two will actually have a baby with Down syndrome.

### Do I need to have the quad marker screen?

Your healthcare provider will recommend that you have a quad marker screen, but it is your decision whether or not to have the test. However, if you have any of the following risk factors, you may strongly want to consider having the test:
- You are age 35 or older when the baby is due
- Your family has a history of birth defects
- You've had a previous child with a birth defect
- You have had insulin-dependent (Type 1) diabetes before your pregnancy

## Genetic Tests

**Ashkenazi Jewish Panel** includes DNA testing for Tay Sachs Disease, Gaucher Disease, Niemann-Pick Disease, Canavan Disease, Bloom Syndrome, Fanconi Anemia, Cystic Fibrosis, and Familial Dysautonomia.

**Cystic Fibrosis (CF) Screening** tests for a genetic disorder that causes problems with breathing and digestion. It is caused by an abnormal gene that is passed from parent to child. There is no cure for CF, but it can be treated. Testing can be done to see if a person carries the gene and if there is a risk of passing it on to a child.

**Hemoglobinopathy Screen** is to identify couples whose children may be at high risk to have an inherited hemoglobinopathy (blood disease). Hemoglobinopathy screening can be performed at any time in pregnancy, but it is most useful when done early in pregnancy (between 10 and 20 weeks).

The above screenings are done for genetic conditions that can be detected by blood tests done ideally before pregnancy or in early pregnancy.

## Genetic Ultrasound

A targeted ultrasound looks for markers associated with Down syndrome and other genetic conditions. An ultrasound may also detect birth defects. This ultrasound is usually performed between 16 weeks and 18 weeks gestation.

## Amniocentesis

This test will detect chromosomal abnormalities. It is an invasive diagnostic test done by inserting a needle into the amniotic fluid. The risk of miscarriage is 1 in 400-700. This diagnostic test is performed between 15 weeks and 23 weeks gestation. This diagnostic test is usually done after an abnormal quad marker screen or offered to moms 35 or older.

# Pregnancy and Sexuality

Many couples wonder medically if sex is safe in pregnancy and if intercourse will harm the baby or the woman. In a pregnancy with no problems, sex is considered safe and healthy. The changes of pregnancy can affect your sexuality and levels of sexual desire for both you and your partner. It is normal for your sex drive to change with the stages of pregnancy as your body image and energy levels change. Your partner's sexual feelings may also change as your pregnancy progresses. Being honest with each other about your needs and emotions is the key to continued intimacy and will help you enjoy a happy and satisfying sexual relationship during pregnancy.

Your comfort should be the most important guide during sex. As pregnancy advances, you and your partner may wish to use positions that do not put pressure on your abdomen, such as lying on your sides together or your partner lying beneath you. If you do have health problems or risk factors during your pregnancy, ask your healthcare provider whether sex will be safe. If certain complications exist, you may be advised to modify your lovemaking, to use a condom during sex, using dental dams for oral sex, or to abstain from having intercourse for your health and the health of your baby.

You should not have sex if you have any bleeding or preterm labor contractions, or if your water breaks before labor.

# Sexually Transmitted Diseases (STDs)

An STD or STI is an infection that you get from someone else by having sexual intercourse. You can get an STD by having vaginal sex (penis in the vagina), anal sex (penis in the rectum), or oral sex (penis in the mouth or mouth on the vagina). After the common cold, STDs are the second most common infections in the United States and Canada. Over a million people each year get STDs.

Anyone who is having sex can get an STD. It is true that if you have had only one partner during your life, you are at less risk. But it is important to remember that you never know for sure if your partner has or has had other partners. Even if you think you're not infected, get checked. You want your baby to have the cleanest bill of health when starting out with his or her new life.

## *What are the Most Common STDs?*

**Chlamydia** is the most common STD in the United States. Most women have no symptoms and do not know when they have Chlamydia. If Chlamydia is not treated, it may cause an infection in the pelvic organs called Pelvic Inflammatory Disease (PID). PID can cause severe pain during the illness and problems getting pregnant (damages fallopian tubes); it can prevent a normal pregnancy in the future. Chlamydia can be cured. Both you and your partner will have to be treated with medication and abstain from intercourse until medication course is completed.

**Trichomoniasis, or "trich,"** is another common STD. You may have a foul-smelling, frothy green discharge, and your genitalia and vagina may itch or burn. Some women have no symptoms. Trich can be cured easily if both you and your partner are treated with medication simultaneously and refrain from intercourse until medication course is completed.

**Herpes** is caused by the Herpes Simplex virus. About one in every 4 adults has herpes. The first outbreak of herpes may cause painful, burning sores on your external genitalia, perineum or buttocks. You can also have lesions in the vagina. Other symptoms include leg pain, headaches, and painful urination. There is no cure, but there are medications that can prevent outbreaks and keep you more comfortable when you have an outbreak. There is Type I (oral) and Type II (genital) herpes simplex virus. Talk to your healthcare provider if you think you may have HSV.

**Genital Warts** may show up as bumpy growths on your perineum/external genitalia that look like cauliflower, which are caused by the Human Papilloma Virus (HPV). About 4 in every 10 adults have this HPV virus. For women, the biggest concern is that certain types of this HPV virus can cause cancer of the cervix. Once you have the HPV virus, your body will carry it forever, and you can pass it to others. Women are advised to have their regular pap smear yearly to screen for cervical cancer. Your yearly pap smear is the only screening test for cervical cancer.

# Pregnancy No-No's

## *Alcohol*

Anything you eat, drink, swallow, or even breathe goes through your blood to your baby through the placenta. All the food and oxygen the baby needs to grow goes through the placenta. Harmful substances such as alcohol, drugs, cigarette smoke, caffeine and the medications you consume also move through the placenta to your baby. Because your baby is so small and growing so quickly, alcohol consumption is very dangerous. The more you drink, the greater the danger to your baby.

Alcohol can cause lifelong health problems for your baby, such as birth defects, learning problems/disabilities, miscarriage, stillbirth, low birth weight and even infant death. Alcohol use can also cause babies to be born with a birth defect called fetal alcohol syndrome (FAS).

Babies with FAS have the following conditions: small heads and heart defects, poor growth in utero and learning problems/disabilities.

It's best not to drink at all when you are pregnant. If you *are* drinking, the time to stop is now. Consult with your healthcare provider for counseling and treatment.

***Oops! I did before I knew I was pregnant!***

The best thing you can do now is to cut alcohol out of your lifestyle. Most healthcare providers agree that a few drinks early on before you know you are pregnant will not adversely affect your baby.

## *Recreational and Illicit Drugs*

Recreational and illicit drugs are harmful no matter who you are. Pregnant women should not use any street/recreational drugs as their babies can develop lifelong problems or may even die.

Cocaine or crack cocaine can cause the placenta to separate from the inside of the uterus before the baby is born (placenta abruption). This can cause severe bleeding that may lead to death for the mother and the baby. Marijuana can cause a baby to be born too early or too small and can produce long-term learning disabilities. It's best not to use drugs at all when you are pregnant. If you need help in stopping the use of drugs, ask your healthcare provider.

***Oops! I did before I knew I was pregnant!***

The best thing you can do now is to cut drugs out of your lifestyle immediately.

## *Smoking*

Smoking during pregnancy affects you and your baby's health before, during and after your baby is born. Nicotine is one of the hardest substances to give up. Ask any smoker who has quit time and time again. Nicotine (the addictive substance in cigarettes), carbon monoxide and numerous other poisons you inhale from a cigarette are carried through your bloodstream and go directly to your baby.

*Smoking while pregnant will:*

- Lower the amount of oxygen available to you and your growing baby
- Increase your baby's heart rate

- Increase the chances of miscarriage and stillbirth
- Increase the risk that your baby is born prematurely and/or born with low birth weight
- Increase your baby's risk of developing respiratory problems

The more cigarettes you smoke per day, the greater your baby's chances of developing these and other health problems. There is no "safe" level of smoking for your baby's health.

### Oops! I did before I knew I was pregnant!

The best thing you can do now is to stop smoking. Most healthcare providers agree that a few cigarettes very early on before you know you are pregnant should not adversely affect your baby.

### What about secondhand smoke exposure?

Secondhand smoke (also called passive smoke or environmental tobacco smoke) is the combination of smoke from a burning cigarette and smoke exhaled by a smoker. The smoke that burns off the end of a cigarette or cigar contains more harmful substances (tar, carbon monoxide, nicotine and others) than the smoke inhaled by the smoker.

If you are regularly exposed to secondhand smoke, you increase your and your baby's risk of developing lung cancer, heart disease, emphysema, allergies, asthma and other health problems.

Babies exposed to secondhand smoke may also develop reduced lung capacity and are at higher risk for sudden infant death syndrome (SIDS). If you continue to smoke after your baby is born, you increase his or her chance of developing certain illnesses and problems, such as:

- Frequent colds
- Bronchitis and pneumonia
- Asthma
- Chronic coughs
- Ear infections
- High blood pressure
- Learning and behavior problems later in childhood

### How can you quit smoking?

There is no one way to quit smoking that works for everyone, since each person has different smoking habits. Here are some tips:

- Make it more difficult to have a quick smoke by hiding your matches, lighters, and ashtrays.
- Take a deep breath and hold it for five to ten seconds whenever you get the urge to smoke.
- Designate your home a non-smoking area.
- Ask people who smoke not to smoke around you.
- Drink less caffeinated beverages; caffeine may stimulate your urge to smoke. Also avoid alcohol, as it also may increase your urge to smoke and can be harmful to your baby.
- Change your habits connected with smoking. If you smoked while driving or when feeling stressed, try other activities to replace smoking.
- Keep mints or gum (preferably sugarless) on hand for those times when you get the urge to smoke.
- Stay active to keep your mind off smoking and help relieve tension; take a walk, exercise, read a book or try a new a hobby.
- Look for support from others. Join a support group or smoking cessation program.
- Do not go to places where many people are smoking such as bars or clubs, and smoking sections of restaurants.

The benefits of not smoking start within days of quitting. After you quit, you and your baby's heart beat will return to normal, and your baby will be less likely to develop breathing problems.

You may have symptoms of withdrawal because your body is used to nicotine, the addictive substance in cigarettes. You may crave cigarettes, be irritable, feel very hungry, cough often, get headaches or have difficulty concentrating.

The withdrawal symptoms are only temporary. They are strongest when you first quit but will go away within 10 to 14 days. When withdrawal symptoms occur, stay in control. Think about your reasons for quitting. Remind yourself that these are signs that your body is healing and getting used to being without cigarettes. Remember that withdrawal symptoms are easier to treat than the major diseases that smoking can cause.

Even after the withdrawal is over, expect periodic urges to smoke. However, these cravings are generally short-lived and will go away whether you smoke or not. Don't Smoke!

If you smoke again (called a relapse) do not lose hope. 75% of those who quit relapse. Most smokers quit three times before they are successful. If you relapse, don't give up! Plan ahead and think about what you will do next time you get the urge to smoke.

### Should I use a nicotine replacement to help me quit?

Nicotine gum and patches are not recommended during pregnancy. They release nicotine into the bloodstream of the smoker who is trying to quit and although these products can reduce withdrawal symptoms and decrease cravings, nicotine is quite toxic and potentially harmful to the fetus (as well as to the infant who is breastfeeding). Therefore, these and any other product containing nicotine are not recommended for the pregnant woman who is trying to quit smoking.

## Excessive Amounts of Caffeine

Some studies have shown that excessive amounts of caffeine (500 mg or more) can increase a woman's chance for miscarriage, while other studies have shown that high levels of caffeine can also increase the chances for a low birth weight baby.

### Oops! I did before I knew I was pregnant!

An average cup of coffee contains 137 mg of caffeine, so a cup or two a day shouldn't have any adverse effect. Just be aware of the total amount of caffeine you are consuming each day (including sodas, tea, and chocolate) and consider switching over to decaf.

## Hot Tubs, Saunas, and Hot Baths

The American College of Obstetricians and Gynecologists (ACOG) recommends that women not raise the body's temperature above 101 degrees F during pregnancy, as this can lead to birth defects. Most hot tubs and saunas are too warm for a pregnant woman, but a warm (not scalding!) bath is perfectly safe.

### Oops! I did before I knew I was pregnant!

Don't stress too much—just stay out of the hot water going forward.

## Cleaning the Cat's Litter Box

Cleaning the cat's litter box is a dirty job but someone's got to do it—during pregnancy, however, that someone shouldn't be you. Cat feces can be infected with toxoplasmosis—a parasite that can cause miscarriage or birth defects.

*Oops! I did before I knew I was pregnant!*

Mention it to your healthcare provider, but don't worry—toxoplasmosis is relatively rare. In the future ask someone else to take care of this dirty job. If you absolutely must change the litter box yourself, be sure to wear plastic gloves and wash your hands after finishing the job.

## Aspirin

Aspirin use in early pregnancy has been linked to increased rates of miscarriage, and in later pregnancy has been shown to increase the risk of placenta abruption.

*Oops! I did before I knew I was pregnant!*

Mention it to your healthcare provider, but it's unlikely that a low dosage of aspirin very early on will cause a problem. Going forward, always check with your health care provider before taking any OTC medications.

## Other Over-the-Counter Medications

Some other OTC medications have been shown to cause problems during pregnancy.

*Oops! I did before I knew I was pregnant!*

Mention it to your healthcare provider, but it's unlikely that a low dosage early on will cause a problem. Again, going forward, always check with your health care provider before taking any OTC medications.

# Foods to Avoid While You are Pregnant

## *Deli Meats*

It's hard to believe that danger could be lurking in something as simple as a deli sandwich, but deli meats can be contaminated with listeria—a bacteria that can cause miscarriage, preterm labor, or infection in your newborn.

***Oops! I did before I knew I was pregnant!***

Symptoms of listeriosis include mild flu-like symptoms, headaches, muscle aches, fever, nausea, and vomiting and typically show up within a few days of consuming the contaminated food. Occasionally it takes a few weeks for symptoms to appear. If you haven't shown any of the symptoms of listeriosis you're probably in the clear. Your best bet is to avoid deli meats altogether, or heat deli meat in the microwave until it is steaming before you take a bite of that sandwich.

## *Raw Meats*

Do not eat any meat that is rotten or raw. Red meat should be cooked to medium or medium well.

## *Sushi*

Uncooked fish and meats may contain parasites and bacteria that could cause harm to your developing baby.

***Oops! I did before I knew I was pregnant!***

Just mention it to your healthcare provider and avoid the raw bar in the future. But you don't have to give up sushi altogether—California rolls and any other types of cooked sushi are perfectly safe.

## Certain types of fish

Certain types of fish, such as shark, swordfish, king mackerel, and tilefish, contain high levels of mercury, which can be damaging to your baby's developing brain and nervous system. Many fish—especially fish that are large, eat other fish, and live a long time—have mercury in them.

Fish may also have dioxins and polychlorinated biphenyls (PCBs). These toxins may also cause problems with the development of your baby's brain and may even cause cancer.

### Oops! I did before I knew I was pregnant!

Don't worry! Just cut high mercury fish out of your diet during the rest of your pregnancy. Please see the lists below.

*You should avoid the following fish completely:*
- Shark
- Swordfish
- King Mackerel
- Tilefish

*You should limit your intake of the following fish:*
- Farmed salmon - Eat no more than 1 meal a month
- Albacore tuna ("white" tuna) - Eat no more than 1 meal a week
- Shrimp, canned light tuna, canned or wild salmon, pollock, canned smoked fish and catfish - Eat no more than 2 meals a week

## Soft Cheeses

The Center for Disease Control has advised pregnant women not to eat soft cheeses such as feta, Brie, Camembert, blue-veined cheeses, queso fresco, queso blanco, and Panela, due to the risk of listeria contamination. Listeriosis can cause miscarriage, preterm labor, or infection in your baby.

If you love dairy products don't despair! You can have all you want of skim or 1% pasteurized milk, hard cheeses, semi-soft cheeses like mozzarella, processed cheese slices, cream cheese, cottage cheese and yogurt made with pasteurized milk.

*Oops! I did before I knew I was pregnant!*

If you haven't developed symptoms of listeriosis (mild flu-like symptoms, headaches, muscle aches, fever, nausea and vomiting) within a few weeks of consumption then the cheese you ate was most likely not contaminated. Going forward, avoid the cheese plate or stick to hard, pasteurized cheeses.

# Common Discomforts

Your body is constantly changing during your pregnancy, which may cause some discomforts. Some of these discomforts may occur in the early weeks of your pregnancy, while others will occur only as you get closer to the birth of your child. Other discomforts may appear early in the pregnancy and go away, only to come back later. This is normal and usually does not mean something is wrong.

Every woman's pregnancy is unique, and some of these changes and discomforts may not affect you. Discuss any concerns about your discomforts with your healthcare provider. Some of the most common discomforts and ways to relieve them are described in the following pages.

## *Abdominal Pain or Discomfort*

Crampy or short, stabbing pains on either side of your abdomen may result from the stretching tissue supporting your growing uterus. The pains are usually noticed upon getting up, changing position, coughing or sneezing; they may be brief or last a couple of hours. These pains may also travel down into your groin, down your thigh and into your leg.

- Change your position or activity until you are comfortable; avoid sharp turns or sudden or sharp movements.
- Apply a hot water bottle, heating pad at moderate temperature or take a warm bath or shower. Be sure the hot water bottle is wrapped with a towel.
- Try massaging the affected area(s).
- Make sure you are drinking enough fluids. You should drink at least 8-10 glasses of fluids/day.
- Contact your healthcare provider if the pain is severe or constant or if you are less than 36 weeks pregnant and you have signs of pre-term or premature labor.

## *Signs Of Preterm (Premature) Contractions*

- More than four to six contractions (tightening of the muscles in the uterus which cause discomfort or a dull ache in the lower abdomen) in an hour, or one contraction every 15 minutes for one hour.
- Regular tightening or pain in your lower back or lower abdominal area.
- Pressure in the pelvis or vagina.
- Menstrual-like cramps.
- Vaginal bleeding.
- Leaking of fluid from the vagina.
- Flu-like symptoms such as nausea, vomiting, or diarrhea.

## *Backaches*

The stable joints of the pelvis begin to loosen up during pregnancy due to the increased amount of progesterone in your body, which allows easier passage for the baby at birth. In addition, your enlarging abdomen throws your body off balance and your center of gravity changes as your pregnancy progresses. As your center of gravity shifts, you may compensate by bringing your shoulders back and arching your back. The curve in your lower back may be exaggerated and result in strained back muscles.

- Wear low-heeled (but not flat) shoes.
- Avoid high-heeled footwear.
- Wear a well fitting and supportive bra.
- Use good posture, not only when standing, but also when sitting.
- Avoid sofas and chairs without good support.
- Avoid excessive weight gain.
- Avoid lifting heavy objects. You should not be lifting any objects greater than 20 pounds without assistance.
- Use proper body mechanics. Squat down with your knees bent when picking up objects instead of bending down at the waist.
- Do not stand for long periods. If you need to stand for long periods, place one foot on a low stool or box with your knee bent. Also, wearing support hose with help provide comfort.

- Support your lower back with a small pillow when sitting or driving for a long period.
- Use a firm mattress for sleeping. If needed, put a board between the mattress and box spring.
- Sleep on your left or right side with a pillow between your legs for support. Body pillows work great for this.
- Apply a hot water bottle (be sure to wrap it in a towel), heating pad at moderate temperature, or take a warm bath or shower.
- Try massage therapy. Ask your healthcare provider for recommendations.
- Perform exercises, as advised by your healthcare provider, to make your back muscles stronger and help relieve the soreness.
- Pelvic rock/pelvic tilt.
- Position is helpful; ask your healthcare provider for more details.
- Chiropractic care can greatly reduce back pain in pregnancy. Your healthcare provider will be glad to recommend a chiropractor who specializes in the treatment of pregnant women and who can explain exercises to relieve back discomfort.

## *Bleeding and Swollen Gums*

The increase in your blood volume and supply of certain hormones may cause tenderness, swelling and bleeding of gums. This swelling is similar to that which takes place in nasal and vaginal mucous membranes. Sensitive gums may become inflamed and bleed. The drain of nutrients for placental and fetal growth can also affect teeth.

- Good preventative care is essential to dental health.
- Take proper care of your teeth and gums. Use a soft toothbrush to brush after every meal. Floss daily.
- See your dentist if you are due for a check-up during your pregnancy. Early in your pregnancy is the ideal time. If you do suspect a problem, consult with your dentist and let him or her know that you are pregnant and what trimester you are presently in.
- Only local anesthetics should be used if necessary for dental work.
- Avoid x-rays unless absolutely necessary and then take special precautions.

- Badly decayed teeth can lead to the spread of infection that may be harmful to you and your baby. There are antibiotics that can be taken during pregnancy if needed. See your dentist with any suspected problems.

## Breast Changes

Your breasts will increase in size as your milk glands become enlarged and the fatty tissues increase, causing breast firmness and tenderness in the first and last few months of pregnancy. Hormonal changes cause increased blood supply to the breast in preparation for milk production. Breasts become tender and the areola (area around the nipple) may become darker. The tenderness usually subsides after the first 3-4 months. The enlargement may continue throughout pregnancy. Bluish veins may also appear as your blood supply increases. Thick fluid called colostrum may leak from your breasts. All of these breast changes are normal.

- Wear a larger, well-supporting bra. Choose cotton bras or those made from other natural fibers. You may even wear a bra at night if it helps with the discomfort.
- Increase your bra size as your breasts become larger. Your bra should fit well without irritating your nipples. Try maternity or nursing bras that provide more support and can be used after pregnancy if you choose to breastfeed.
- Tuck a cotton handkerchief or nursing pads into each bra cup to absorb leaking fluid.
- Clean your breasts with warm water only; *do not use soap or other products.*

## Complexion Problems

Hormonal changes cause an increased secretion of oils on your face.
- Drink plenty of water (at least 64 oz. per day).
- Maintain good nutrition including fresh foods.
- Wash your face with a gentle cleanser.
- Avoid greasy creams and makeup. Moisturize with a gentle face cream if your skin gets dry, especially in the winter months.

## *Constipation*

The hormonal changes in pregnancy slow intestinal activity and cause fluid to shift to the tissues. Vitamins and iron supplements may cause constipation (difficulty passing stool or incomplete or infrequent passage of hard stools). Pressure on your rectum from your uterus may also cause constipation.

- Drink plenty of fluids; preferably water (at least 64 ounces daily!).
- Include fresh fruits and fruit juices in your diet. Prune juice is often effective, tastes great over ice!
- Include more fiber in your diet (whole grains, bran cereal, or bran muffins).
- Increase exercise to increase intestinal activity. Walking a mile per day can be helpful for constipation as well as for a general feeling of well-being.
- Drink warm liquids, especially in the morning upon arising.
- Set a regular time for bowel movements; avoid straining when having a bowel movement. Take your time!
- Take alfalfa tablets (you can get these at a health food store; start with one daily and work up to 2-3 after each meal, 6-9 total. If you experience loose stools, cut back on the number of tablets. (Alfalfa tablets also help to boost your blood count and increase milk production.)
- Talk to your healthcare provider before using mild laxatives, stool softeners and/or glycerin suppositories.

## *Difficulty Sleeping*

Finding a comfortable resting position can become difficult as your pregnancy progresses and your uterus enlarges.

- Avoid sleep medications.
- Take a warm bath or shower before bedtime.
- Drink some warm milk at bedtime or sleepy time herbal tea.
- Use extra pillows for support while sleeping. Lying on your side, place a pillow under your head, abdomen, behind your back and between your knees to prevent muscle strain and help you get the rest you need. You will probably feel better lying on your left side; this improves circulation of the blood throughout your body.
- Adjust fluid intake: increase during the day, decrease in the evening.

- Eat something high in protein before bedtime.
- Try meditation, relaxation, breathing, or massage.
- Skullcap tincture, a natural herb; (1-10 drops in hot water).

## Dizziness or Faintness

During pregnancy, the enlarging uterus, along with hormonal changes, can cause blood to collect in the lower extremities. Getting up too quickly may cause a temporary decrease in blood pressure and resulting dizziness. Low blood sugar or a lack of adequate iron may also contribute.

- Get up slowly, especially from a lying down position. Turning on your side before sitting up from a lying position will help.
- Avoid wearing tight clothing, especially constricting hose that will impede blood flow.
- Move slowly when standing from a sitting position; avoid sudden movements.
- Carry a snack with you at all times to avoid blood sugar drops.
- If you have persistent dizzy spells or you faint, call your healthcare provider or nurse-midwife immediately.

## Emotional Instability or Moodiness

Hormonal changes may cause you to feel moody, sad, or irritable. If this is your first baby, you and your partner will need to adjust to a change in family dynamics. This transition can be frightening at times. If this is not your first baby, older siblings must also adjust. If this pregnancy was unplanned, you may be faced with sudden decisions and adaptations. All of these situations can be both happy and stressful. Give yourself time to adjust. Open communication between you and your partner is essential.

## Fatigue or Sleepiness

Your body is working very hard to manufacture a placenta, adjust to the physiological changes in pregnancy, and help your new baby grow. Is it normal to feel tired? Absolutely! Changes in the levels of your hormones and emotional changes play a significant role in these symptoms.

- Get plenty of rest; try to nap during the day or go to bed earlier at night.

- Don't plan late nights out for a while. Maintain a regular schedule when possible but pace your activities; balance activity with rest when needed.
- Exercise daily to increase your energy level.
- You will have more energy when your body has adjusted to pregnancy and the placenta is essentially complete.

## *Frequent Urination*

During the first trimester, hormonal changes and the enlarging uterus affect your urinary system. As the uterus expands upward, pressure on your bladder will decrease. Softening of the lower part of the uterus and enlargement causes it to become more anteflexed (bent forward) in the first trimester. Later, it will grow upward and take the pressure off the bladder (until the last trimester when the abdomen becomes crowded by the greatly enlarged uterus). Urination at night, which interrupts sleep, is caused in part by the improved venous return, which occurs when lying down.

- Plan your day for frequent bathroom breaks.
- Avoid tight fitting underwear, pants or panty hose.
- Do Kegel exercises to strengthen pelvic floor muscles.
- Don't drink within 1-2 hours of bedtime for a better night's sleep.
- Limit caffeine intake, especially in the later part of the day.
- Contact your healthcare provider if your urine burns or stings. This can be a sign of a urinary tract infection and should be treated immediately.

## *Urinary Tract Infection*

A Urinary Tract Infection or UTI is a frequent urge to urinate accompanied by burning and/or sharp lower abdominal pain. The pressure of the uterus on the bladder may prevent complete emptying, allowing urine to stagnate and bacteria to multiply. Increased vaginal discharge (normal in pregnancy) may collect and work its way into the urethra.

- Drink plenty of fluids, particularly water. Unsweetened citrus and cranberry juices may be helpful, but avoid coffee, tea, alcohol, and cola drinks.
- Empty your bladder just before and after sexual intercourse.
- Each time you urinate, take time to be sure your bladder is completely empty.

- Wear cotton-crotch underwear and avoid wearing tight clothing or panty hose.
- Keep vaginal and perineal area clean.
- Wash daily, but avoid perfumed soaps, powders, and bubble baths.
- Always wipe front to back!
- Maintain good nutrition to keep your immune system functioning well.
- Always finish prescribed medications and take according to directions.

## *Headaches*

The stress of adjusting to pregnancy and to hormonal changes may aggravate headaches. Sinus headaches may be due to congestion of mucous membranes caused by pregnancy hormones. Fluctuations in blood sugar levels, caused by eating high-carbohydrate foods or not eating regular meals, may also contribute to headaches. Sleeplessness is also a factor. Stay well hydrated!

- Apply ice pack to your forehead or the back of your neck.
- Rest, sit or lie quietly in a low-lit room. Close your eyes and try to release the tension in your back, neck and shoulders.
- Most headaches in pregnancy are of the tension variety. Consider chiropractic treatments for head, neck, back, hip and leg discomfort (your healthcare provider will be happy to recommend a chiropractor who specializes in the treatment of pregnant women).
- Eat regularly and try to get enough rest. Try including high-protein snacks in your diet. Relaxation and quiet can work wonders!
- Steam from a warm shower may relieve sinus congestion. You may take Tylenol for an isolated headache. Sudafed is also appropriate, according to package instructions, for congestion.
- Ask for advice before taking any other medications for your headache.
- Contact your healthcare provider if: you have nausea with your headache, if your headache is severe and is not relieved with these measures, or if you have blurry vision, double vision or blind spots.
- Contact your healthcare provider if your are experiencing persistent headaches after 28 weeks of gestation or a headache accompanied by swelling in hands, feet or legs, blurred or double vision, or heartburn-type pain.

## *Heartburn, Indigestion, or Flatulence*

Heartburn (indigestion) is a burning feeling that starts in the stomach and seems to rise to the throat. The rising levels of progesterone during pregnancy slow down the digestive tract. This slowing of food digestion may make you uncomfortable; however, it allows increased absorption of nutrients necessary for proper growth and development of your baby. Also, your enlarged uterus can crowd your stomach, intestines and bladder, pushing stomach acids upward, which can cause additional heartburn.

- Eat slowly and chew thoroughly. Eliminate foods that cause discomfort (highly seasoned foods, fatty foods, fried food, processed meats, chocolate, coffee, and carbonated beverages).
- Eat several small meals each instead of three large meals.
- Drink warm, herbal, decaffeinated tea or warm water with lemon.
- Do not lie down or even recline for at least 90 minutes after eating.
- Avoid wearing tight clothing and avoid bending at the waist.
- Avoid greasy foods; these depress motility of stomach and secretion of gastric juices needed for digestion.
- Avoid very cold foods with meals.
- Avoid spicy foods, orange juice or tomato-based foods.
- Drink ½ glass of club soda or mineral water after a meal.
- Drink cultured milk, skim milk and/or eat low-fat ice cream.
- Take a few alfalfa tablets after meals; it may help neutralize acidity.
- Have a small peppermint candy after meals.
- Avoid heavy or full meals before bedtime.
- Try papaya enzymes with Chlorophyll as directed on the package.
- Try taking a natural enzyme supplement such as Beano® with first bite of food.
- Sleep with your head elevated 6 inches or place pillows under your shoulders to prevent stomach acids from rising into your chest.
- Practice deep, slow breathing and a regular method of relaxation.
- Try not to combine eating with other activities (e.g., watching TV, driving or working).
- If these methods do not provide relief, you may take Tums occasionally. (Do not overuse!!)

- Do not take antacids that are high in sodium, such as Alka Seltzer or sodium bicarbonate.
- Antacids containing magnesium may cause diarrhea, and those with aluminum are associated with constipation. Be sure to read the labels.

## *Hemorrhoids and Varicose Veins*

Hemorrhoids are simply varicose veins of the rectum and affect 20-50% of all pregnant women. Increased blood volume and pressure from the enlarging uterus contribute to varicose veins in the lower half of the body. Constipation compounds the problem. Itching and bleeding of the hemorrhoids may also occur.

Varicose veins in your legs can also become large or swollen for the same reasons. Although varicose veins are usually hereditary, below are some preventive tips along with tips regarding hemorrhoids:

- Do not self-diagnose rectal bleeding. Allow your healthcare provider to evaluate the problem.
- If you know you have hemorrhoids, avoid constipation. Do not strain during a bowel movement.
- Sleep on your side to avoid putting extra pressure on rectal veins.
- Avoid sitting for long periods of time. Get up and move around often.
- Rest periods with legs elevated.
- Engage in mild exercise and walking.
- Control weight gain.
- Wear maternity abdominal support belt.
- Take vitamin B6 for swelling.
- Increase protein intake.
- Apply ice packs or cold compresses to the area or take a warm tub bath a few times a day to provide relief. Tucks pads are also beneficial.
- Avoid tight fitting underwear, pants or pantyhose.
- Perform Kegel exercises to improve circulation in the area (please ask your healthcare provider for information on Kegel exercises). Use Kegel exercises for vulvar varicosities. These are much like varicose veins in the legs except they appear in the area of the vulva.
- Keep the perineal area very clean.

- Lie down on your side several times during the day in a right angle position.
- Use astringent or Epsom salt compresses.
- Try topical anesthetics such as Anusol or Preparation H.
- Try bed rest with hips and lower extremities elevated—either on pillows or knee-chest position.
- Avoid remaining in any position that might restrict the circulation in your legs (e.g., crossing your legs while sitting).
- Elevate your legs and feet while sitting.
- Exercise regularly.
- Wear support stockings - put on before rising.
- Avoid knee high leg wear.
- Provide physical support for vulvar varicosities—pads or belts (use a peri-pad which is similar to a maxi pad with a support panty).

## Increased Fetal Activity

As the fetus grows, his/her activity becomes much more noticeable. Arms and legs become stronger and you may notice larger, "rolling" movements as well as kicks and hiccups (felt as regular little spasms in abdomen). Some of these movements may be uncomfortable or you may feel "bruised" on the inside of your abdomen. In your last couple of weeks of pregnancy, you may notice that movements trigger a contraction or vice versa.

Be reassured that your baby's movements are a sign of well-being. You should be feeling significant movement every day after fetal activity is well established. Moist heat to areas of discomfort may help, but you may just have to tolerate a very active baby.

If you do not feel any fetal movement for a better part of a day, please notify your healthcare provider so that they can evaluate your baby's well-being.

## Leg Cramps

Pressure from your growing uterus can cause leg cramps or sharp pains down your legs, especially in the calf area.

- Be sure to eat and drink foods and beverages rich in calcium (e.g., milk, broccoli, spinach, cheese).
- Wear comfortable, low-heeled shoes.

- Try wearing support hose, BUT avoid any leg wear that is too tight and constricting.
- Elevate your legs when possible; avoid crossing your legs.
- Exercise daily; stretch your legs before going to bed.
- Avoid lying on your back: the weight of your body and the pressure of your enlarged uterus can slow the circulation in your legs, causing cramps.
- Gently stretch any muscle that becomes cramped by straightening your leg, flexing your foot and pulling your toes toward you.
- Try massaging the cramp, or apply heat or a hot water bottle (wrapped in a towel) to sore area.
- Sleep with lower legs elevated slightly on a pillow.
- Increase B vitamins - meats, whole grains, nuts, wheat germ, brewer's yeast, nutritional yeast, eggs, and green veggies.
- Decrease phosphorus intake – soft drinks, processed foods.

## Nasal Congestion

High levels of estrogen in pregnancy bring increased blood flow to mucous membranes, causing them to soften and swell, giving you that "stuffy nose" feeling like you have a "cold."

- Apply a warm, wet washcloth to your cheeks, eyes and nose to reduce congestion.
- Drink plenty of fluids (at least 8 to 10 glasses of fluids/day) to thin mucous.
- Elevate your head with an extra pillow while sleeping to prevent mucous from blocking your throat.
- A cool mist vaporizer or humidifier will help to add moisture to the air in the winter months.
- If you must blow your nose frequently, do so gently to avoid damage to nasal membranes.
- Avoid nasal sprays and medications. They can aggravate your symptoms.

## Nausea or Vomiting ("Morning Sickness")

Nausea can occur at any time of the day but may be worse in the morning when your stomach is empty (hence the term "morning sickness") or if you are not eating enough or frequently enough. They key is to keep something in your stomach frequently to avoid that "green" feeling. Nausea is a result of hormonal changes in your body and most often occurs early in pregnancy until your body adjusts to the increased production of hormones.

*Before you go to bed:*
- Be sure to have plenty of fresh air in the room where you sleep. The odor of soiled clothes and other household scents in the room where you sleep may upset your stomach.
- Place some dry cereal or dry bread within reach of your bed to make it easy to reach. You could also try toast, dry biscuits, uncooked oatmeal, ready-to-eat cereals, or crackers. Chew slowly if need be, taking little bites so your stomach will settle.
- Try eating a high-protein snack such as lean meat or cheese before going to bed (protein takes longer to digest).

*Before you get up in the morning:*
- East some of the dry bread, cereal or crackers. A small amount of jelly may make it taste better.
- Do not use butter or margarine.

*When you get up:*
- Get up very slowly; take several minutes while changing positions.
- Avoid sudden movements when getting out of bed.

*When you cook breakfast:*
- Eat some more dry bread, cereal or crackers a little while after you get up and before you cook breakfast.
- Have a window open while you cook breakfast to get rid of the odor of cooking foods.

*For nausea during the day:*
- Eat several small meals a day instead of three large ones. You are more likely to feel nauseated when your stomach is empty. Eat slowly and chew your food completely.
- Avoid spicy, fried or greasy foods. If you are bothered by strong smells, eat foods cold or at room temperature and avoid odors that bother you.
- Do not drink fluids or eat soups at mealtime. Wait at least one hour after eating your meal to drink fluids.

- Avoid large amounts of fluids at one time.
- If you are thirsty, try eating chips of ice.
- Sometime during the day, you will find you can eat a regular meal. Be sure not to overeat at this time.

*Foods to Avoid:*
- Fatty and greasy foods may upset the stomach. Eat very little or none of the following foods: butter, margarine, gravy, bacon, salt, pork, oils, mayonnaise, salad dressings, pie crusts, pastries.
- Highly seasoned foods, such as those cooked with garlic, onion, pepper, chili, and other spices may upset your stomach. Eat lightly seasoned foods.
- Do not eat foods that give you gas.

*Between Meals:*
- Drink small sips of liquids frequently between meals. Drink milk, water, fruit juices, coffee, tea and soups between meals *only*. Herbal teas, such as raspberry leaf, chamomile, spearmint, peppermints or ginger root may help.
- When you feel nauseated, drink a *small* amount of these fluids: cool, carbonated beverages, clear fruit juices, such as apple or grape juice. Popsicles or frozen fruit bars may be tolerated best. Above all, eat or drink what sounds good to you.

*Other Recommendations:*
- Sea bands or acupressure wristbands, which are frequently used for motion sickness, are helpful for morning sickness. These bands can be purchased at your local drug store. Your pharmacist or healthcare provider can help you with correct placement of the bands. Simple instructions are provided in the package insert too.
- Carry sourball candy in your pocket to suck on between meals.
- Candy known as Fireballs can also help with nausea.
- Eat anything ginger. Ginger cookies, ginger tea, and ginger ale. You can find this spice in the health food or vitamin stores. As a supplement, purchase the 250 mg capsules.
- Take papaya tablets. Talk to your healthcare provider about recommended dosages.

If your vomiting is constant or you continue to vomit for 24 hours or more, you cannot keep anything down (fluids or food), or feel weak and dizzy, call your healthcare provider immediately. This can cause dehydration and should be treated right away. You may need intravenous hydration at this point.

## Shortness of Breath

Hormonal changes may cause a decreased tolerance to carbon dioxide and brief feelings of breathlessness. Later in pregnancy, the enlarging uterus presses upward against the diaphragm and allows less room for lung expansion.

- Be reassured that this feeling is normal as long as it is not associated with chest pain or heaviness. In later pregnancy, straighten your posture, sleep with two pillows, and avoid overexertion. Lie on your left side if the feeling is uncomfortable.
- Raise your arm over your head (this lifts the rib cage and allows you to breathe in more air) and take some slow, deep breaths.
- Notify your healthcare provider if significant discomfort is present or breathlessness seems to persist or worsen.

## Stretch Marks

Stretch marks are a type of scar tissue that forms when the skin's normal elasticity is not enough for the stretching required during pregnancy. Stretch marks usually appear on the abdomen and can also appear on the breasts, buttocks, or thighs. The skin is stretching across the enlarging abdomen and breasts and may also cause itching. While they will not disappear completely, stretch marks will fade after birth. Stretch marks affect the surface under the skin and are usually not preventable.

- Be sure your diet contains enough sources of the nutrients needed for health skin (especially Vitamins C and E).
- Keep your abdominal skin from drying out. Use Aveeno bath soaks. You may try Vitamin E oil on the abdomen, but expensive lotions and creams will probably not be effective in reducing stretch marks.
- Exercise daily.
- Avoid excessive weight gain and/or rapid weight gain

## *Swelling in the Feet and Legs (Edema)*

The enlarging uterus puts pressure on the blood vessels carrying blood from the lower body, causing fluid retention that results in swelling (edema) in the legs and feet. Prolonged standing, constrictive clothing, hot weather, and excessive salt intake in your diet aggravate swelling.

- Try not to stay on your feet for long periods.
- Avoid standing in one place.
- Drink plenty of fluids (at least 8-10 glasses of fluids a day). Mild exercise and increased fluid intake have a positive diuretic effect.
- Avoid foods high in salt (sodium). Do not take diuretic medication or restrict salt intake beyond reason.
- Rest with legs and feet elevated while sitting (above heart level), or rest on your left side to decrease edema in your legs and to help increase blood flow to your kidneys.
- Avoid crossing your legs. Avoid wearing tight shoes. Choose supportive shoes with low, wide heels.
- Keep your diet rich in protein; too little protein can cause fluid retention.
- If swelling is noticed in hands or face or is accompanied by a headache, blurred vision, or heartburn-type pain, please notify your healthcare provider immediately.

## *Increased Vaginal Discharge*

Normal increased estrogen in pregnancy and increased blood supply causes increased production of vaginal mucous. Normal vaginal discharge is white or clear, non-irritating, odorless and may look yellow when dry on your underwear or panty liner.

- Wear cotton underwear or brands made from other natural fibers. Change underwear frequently or wear a panty-liner (unscented)
- Wash perineal area carefully. Clean the vaginal area with mild soap and water. Wipe yourself from front to back.
- Avoid tight-fitting jeans or pants.
- *DO NOT douche! It* is possible you can introduce air into your circulatory system or break your bag of waters in later pregnancy. It also washes away your good bacteria and makes you prone to bacterial infections.

- Avoid the use of harsh soaps or powders.
- If you notice a change in the color or consistency of the discharge or if it is accompanied by itching, burning, cramping, redness or an odor, please notify your healthcare provider. These symptoms may indicate an infection, which could be harmful to your baby. Most vaginal infections can be safely treated with medication after the first trimester of pregnancy.

## Conclusion

This section may have been scary, telling you all the things not to do and what to avoid. It's ok. You know now! This book is your guideline. We're here as your resource.

# First Trimester

That first pregnancy test finally came back positive, but you're still wondering, am I really pregnant? Are they sure? Am I sure?

*Yes.* Welcome to feeling more tired than you've ever felt before! Rest. You're going to hear more opinions than you've ever dreamed of. Ignore all the negative things. Listen only to the positive. Research only when your intuition tells you that you need to know more about a topic of concern.

Whether you're excited about this pregnancy, scared to death, or still in denial, you are in for the most amazing experience of your life. You're going to notice every little difference in your body, every twinge, every shift. You're going to notice the strangest smells and start watching how small children and their parents interact everywhere you go.

One of the most important aspects of the first trimester is keeping your energy levels up. And trust us, that's no small feat! Pregnancy typically conjures up thoughts of fatigue and exhaustion—and while nearly every pregnant woman experiences a decrease in energy at some point during pregnancy, there are ways to boost energy levels and keep you moving right along until you give birth.

## First Trimester Development

| Timeframe | Development |
| --- | --- |
| *Conception to Six Weeks* | For the first eight weeks, your developing baby is called an embryo. |
| | The baby is growing inside a sac of amniotic fluid (bag of waters). |
| | Hereditary characteristics, such as eye and hair color were determined when the sperm met the egg. |
| | The brain, nervous system, heart and lungs are forming. |
| | Tiny spots for ears, eyes and nose are showing. |
| | The arm and leg buds are forming. |
| | Your baby will be about ¼ inch to 1 inch long and will weigh less than 1 ounce. |

| Seven to Eleven Weeks | This is a key time in your baby's development. |
|---|---|
| | All the major body organs and systems are formed though not completely developed |
| | The heart is beating. The baby's heartbeat is 120 to 160 beats per minute. |
| | The stomach, liver, and kidneys are developing. |
| | The umbilical cord has formed; it will deliver nutrients from mother to baby until cut at the birth of your child. |
| | Eyes and ears are in a critical time of growth. |
| | Facial features are forming. The head is large, since the brain grows faster than the other organs. |
| | Cartilage, skin, and muscles are starting to shape your baby's body. |
| | Fingers, toes, fingernails, ears, ankles, and wrists are forming. |
| | After eight weeks the embryo is called a fetus. The baby is still too tiny for you to feel movement. |
| | Your baby will weigh about ½ ounce to 1 ounce and will be about 2 ¼ inches long. |
| Twelve to Fifteen Weeks | If you could see inside the uterus, the sex of the baby would be easy to identify. |
| | The ears, arms, hands, fingers, legs, feet and toes are formed. |
| | The neck is well shaped and can support the head. |
| | Reflex movements allow your baby's elbows to bend, legs to kick and fingers to form a fist. |
| | Your baby's vocal cords are formed. |
| | Blood is now traveling through the umbilical cord to the baby and will continue to do so until the cord is cut at delivery. |
| | The face is looking more and more human each day as the eyes begin to move closer together instead of being on the sides of the head and the ears move to a normal position. |
| | The intestines move farther into the baby's body; the liver begins to produce insulin. |
| | Your baby begins to practice inhaling and exhaling movements. |
| | Your baby will weigh about ¼ pound and will be about 2¼ inches long. |

**Table 3. Fetal Development in the First Trimester.**

# Six Ways to Boost Your Energy during Pregnancy

Here are six ways to increase your energy levels and stay happier and healthier in the beginning of your pregnancy and beyond:

## #1: Exercise

Exercise is important to a healthy pregnancy and a common factor among pregnant women who say they felt energetic during their pregnancy. If you can commit a little time to physical activity it can give you a huge energy payoff. But just what sorts of exercise can keep your energy up? Just about anything that gets you on your feet and moving is beneficial and here are just a few ideas to get you started. Low impact is best while you are pregnant.

- **Get Moving**: With your healthcare provider's permission, make it a habit to engage in physical activity each day. Take a brief walk outside during the day or perform some light yoga stretches at lunch or while you cook dinner. Your body will thank you!
- **Don't just sit and watch TV**, get moving! Rather than just sitting to watch your favorite TV show, use those 30 minutes for exercise. You can walk on the treadmill or use a stationary bike as you watch. You can sit on your exercise ball. This is also a good time to do some light weights or an exercise band in front of the TV to keep your muscles toned. Exercise will energize your body and increase the blood flow which nourishes your body.
- **Making Exercise Fun**: Make exercise something you look forward to by picking activities you enjoy. You aren't limited to treadmills and toning exercises all the time. Dance to your favorite radio station or put on your favorite dance CD, for example.
- **Find Someone To Exercise With You:** Having someone to exercise with can make it more fun. Find another pregnant mom who you can share a nice walk through a park with. Or hire a prenatal fitness trainer to help motivate you and help you exercise in a safe and healthy way.

## *#2: Getting Enough (Quality) Sleep*

We are always striving to fit as many things as possible into our day. Often, in this pursuit to get everything done, we put sleep at the bottom of the list. Making time for sleep is essential to feeling alert and ready to take on the day, during pregnancy and even after birth. One of the keys to maintaining good energy levels is getting at least eight to nine hours of quality sleep a night. We know this might seem impossible at best, but do what you can to making quality sleep a high priority. Your changing body will appreciate it!

Another key to a good night's sleep is your sleeping position. The best position for you to sleep during pregnancy is on your side. If possible, sleeping on your left side is best. Sleeping on your left side will increase the amount of blood and nutrients that reach the placenta and your baby. Placing a pillow between your legs and keeping your legs bent at the knees will help too. Pillows in front and behind your back will help with comfort also.

## *#3: Eat Healthy!*

Eating healthy provides many benefits and is so important for your body and mind! Energy is just one of those benefits you will get from eating those foods which are packed with nutrients and energy-boosting substances. As your pregnancy continues, and your baby grows, there will be demands on your body that can only be met with a healthy diet.

For example, you can boost your body's healing capabilities by eating foods containing vitamin B6, which helps the body produce serotonin, creating a calming effect and has been shown to help keep morning sickness at bay. We all understand nothing can sap energy faster than morning sickness! Vitamin B6 is found in animal sources like chicken, but is also available in non-animal sources such as sweet potatoes, bell peppers, garlic and bananas.

Another idea is to add nuts such as cashews, almonds and walnuts to your diet. These nuts are rich in protein and contain magnesium, which is a mineral that plays a vital role in converting sugar into energy to keep you moving.

Check out our Nutrition section starting on page 83 where we provide an overview of foods that are healthy and pack an energetic punch!

## *#4: Drink Plenty of Water!*

Along with your food intake, it is important to make sure you drink plenty of water. All chemical processes involve energy metabolism and drinking plenty of water can help you feel more energetic. Pregnant women, especially, should drink the recommended eight ounce, eight to ten glasses of water a day to keep healthy, hydrated and maintain energy.

## *#5: Getting the Proper Supplementation*

No matter how conscientious you are about eating all the healthy foods needed for a healthy pregnancy, there can still be nutritional deficiencies. Your prenatal vitamin is an important way to boost energy and avoid lows, giving your body the extra nutrients you and your baby need.

During pregnancy, your developing baby takes all the nutrients it requires first, and you get what is left over. As the baby grows, energy requirements continue to increase each trimester and you may find it difficult to make healthy food choices to keep up with the increased caloric and energy requirements. It becomes critically important you are getting all the nutritional requirements to support fetal development and growth, and your body requirements to support maternal tissues (e.g., placenta and breast), metabolism and reproduction changes.

It is no wonder we feel so exhausted during pregnancy with all these additional demands made on our bodies! Every pregnant mom will quickly notice the increase energy expenditures during pregnancy. Prenatal vitamins are a great way to help meet the nutritional needs for a healthy pregnancy. Giving your body the nutrients it needs is a great way to make sure you have the extra energy you (and your baby) need.

## *#6: Relaxation and Maintaining Calm*

Pregnancy can be a stressful time, but it's important to learn how to relax, and both you and your baby will benefit. When you are stressed, your body makes physical and chemical changes to try to protect it. If Mom feels calm, relaxed and happy, these feelings will be passed on to your baby. Having a calm and collected mind is vital to staying healthy during pregnancy. A few ways to keep the peace include:

- **Meditation:** Closing your eyes, and focusing on a single image or thought for a few minutes a day can reduce blood pressure, boost the immune system, and provide you with more energy. Meditation is the art of silencing the mind. When the mind is silent, concentration is increased and we experience inner peace in the midst of worldly turmoil. If you find it hard to meditate, try taking deep breaths for a two-minute interval. By slowly and deeply inhaling and exhaling, you calm the body and mind, and restore energy.

- **Take time for you:** Taking time each day for yourself can significantly lower stress and keep your energy levels high. Taking that much needed nap can restore expended energy. Listen to your favorite music or indulge in that good book you've wanted to read. Whatever your pleasure, set aside time to enjoy it. Taking just a few short breaks a day can make a difference in helping to control stress.

- **Take time for your family and friends:** You and your partner are in this journey together; make time for your partner during these busy nine months. Plan that special date night out, a movie night in or game night with friends. It is important to take time for friends and family to keep you connected and they will love being able to share this special time in your life.

---

### Energy Boost

Having, building or sustaining high energy levels during pregnancy doesn't have to be a something you only wish for. By listening to your body, taking care of yourself, and following these tips, you will experience more energy so you can fully enjoy your pregnancy and the planning process for your baby's arrival.

---

# Medical Considerations

Be prepared to spend a lot of time in your healthcare provider's office over the next nine months. This section is to help you navigate those first key visits.

## *Prenatal Care: Your Initial Prenatal Visit*

Regular appointments with your healthcare provider throughout your pregnancy are essential to ensure the health of you and your baby. Prenatal care includes education in pregnancy and childbirth, breastfeeding, plus counseling and support. Your prenatal visits are family-focused and your healthcare provider, whether you choose a nurse midwife or a physician, should strongly encourage family participation in all prenatal visits and education.

Frequent visits with your healthcare provider allow you and your family to follow the progress of your baby's development. Your visits also give you the opportunity to ask questions. Be sure to write down your questions as they come to mind in between visits so you can address them at your next visit. It's okay to bring a list to your visit to have all of your questions and concerns addressed.

Your initial prenatal visit will be the longest visit of your prenatal care. Your healthcare provider determines your general health with a comprehensive history and physical examination. He or she will discuss the risk factors, which may affect your pregnancy.

*Also during this visit your healthcare provider will:*
• Determine your due date
• Explore the medical history of family members on your side of the family and also your partner's family history
• Determine if you have any pregnancy risk factors based on your age, health and/or personal and family history

Your healthcare provider will discuss with you in detail your previous pregnancies, surgeries, medical history and possible exposure to any contagious diseases or environmental hazards. Be sure to give your provider a full run-down of the prescriptions, medications and supplements you are taking. This includes any herbal supplements. Be as complete as possible about everything in your personal and family history, you and your baby deserve the best care, and your information can help provide it.

## *Comprehensive Physical Examination*

Your healthcare provider will perform a comprehensive physical examination, including a pelvic examination. Before your exam, your blood pressure and weight will be obtained along with a clean-catch urine sample for a urinalysis and culture.

During your pelvic examination, a pap smear may be obtained to screen for cervical cancer if you have not had one in the past year. In addition, a bimanual internal exam using both hands for simultaneous internal and external examination will be performed to determine the size and position of your uterus and your pelvis. This exam will also note any abnormalities of the uterus, ovaries, or fallopian tubes.

Your provider may listen to the baby's heartbeat with a special instrument called a Doppler, which uses ultrasound waves. A Doppler usually cannot detect a baby's heartbeat before eleven weeks of pregnancy.

## *Laboratory Tests*

All soon to be mothers go through a series of lab tests. Some require fasting beforehand. For the tests that do require you to fast, a good tip is to schedule those as early as possible in the morning and bring a quick snack to eat afterward so you're not tempted to stop for fast food!

Here's a brief overview of early pregnancy lab tests:
- **Complete Blood Count (CBC)** – screens for blood problems such as anemia
- **RPR** – screens for syphilis (a sexually transmitted infection)
- **Rubella** – tests for immunity (protection) against German measles
- **HbsAg** – tests for Hepatitis B (liver infection)
- **Urinalysis, with culture if indicated** – tests for kidney disease or bladder infections
- **HIV Screening**
- **Type and screen** – determines your blood type and Rh factor (an antigen or protein on the surface of blood cells that causes an immune system response. You can either be Rh positive or Rh negative. If the mother's blood does NOT contain the Rh factor, it is considered to be Rh negative (Rh-). If your blood is Rh- and your baby's blood is Rh+, your body may produce antibodies to protect itself from this "foreign" substance.

Other laboratory tests may be needed depending on your medical and/or your family history, or your individual special needs.

## *Schedule of Prenatal Visits*

The schedule of prenatal visits will depend on any special circumstances or risk factors you may have.

*Generally, it is recommended to have follow-up prenatal visits with your healthcare provider as follows:*
- Every 4 weeks until 28 weeks gestation
- Every 2 weeks from 28 weeks to 36 weeks gestation
- Weekly from 36 weeks until birth

During your follow-up prenatal visits with your healthcare provider, your weight and blood pressure will be checked and a urine sample will be tested for sugar and protein. Your abdomen will be measured to follow the growth of your baby. The baby's heartbeat will also be checked (usually after 11 weeks via Doppler).

During the last month of your prenatal visits, emphasis will be placed on the labor and birth of your child, your desires in labor, and your expectations. At your 32 to 36 week visit, your healthcare provider will encourage you to think about these things along with a birth plan. If you're like those of us writing this book, you'll have your birth plan well under way far in advance of this appointment. Discussion of your birth plan with your provider will be done at one of these follow-up visits to address your concerns, desires, and expectations.

# Concerns about Depression in Pregnancy

Pregnancy isn't always a happy time. It can often be filled with feelings of stress, anxiety, ambivalence, and worry. Although pregnancy has long been viewed as a period of well-being that has protected women against psychiatric diseases, approximately 10-20% of women will struggle with symptoms of depression during their pregnancy. About 10% of women develop major depression.

Depression is a mood disorder that makes you feel deep sadness and can cause extreme dips in your mood that can interfere with your daily activities such as sleeping, eating, or working. Depression is a fairly common condition but when depression occurs during pregnancy there is increased concern about your health and the health of your baby.

Depression is actually caused by a number of different factors. First and foremost, depression seems to be linked to a change in the levels of chemicals in the brain that control mood such as serotonin, dopamine and norepinephrine. When these chemicals become disrupted it can lead to depression. Let's look at what happens when there is a change in the balance of serotonin. Serotonin regulates happiness and affects your ability to function emotionally, and mentally as well as physically. So when there is an imbalance, all these functions are affected.

The rapid changes in hormone levels during pregnancy are believed to be what triggers depression in some women. Depression can also be triggered by personal factors such as stressful events, financial troubles, interpersonal conflict, or by psychological and emotional factors as well.

## *Predisposition for Depression During Pregnancy*

*There a number of factors that affect your predisposition to depression:*
- A history of depression, especially if you have stopped taking antidepressant medication while trying to conceive, or if you suffer from PMDD (Premenstrual Dysphoric Disorder, a severe type of premenstrual syndrome or PMS) or a family history of depression
- Limited social support
- Substance abuse (alcohol, tobacco, drugs)
- Stress or anxiety
- Ambivalence about pregnancy
- Marital conflict
- Poverty
- Childhood trauma, like death or illness of a parent or sibling
- Constant fatigue
- Uncharacteristic behavior
- Thoughts of self-harm or suicide

Depression during pregnancy not only affects you but can also affect your baby. Research has found that women with symptoms of depression are more likely to experience a preterm birth. It has also been shown that the greater the severity of depression symptoms, the greater the likelihood of an early or preterm birth.

Another problem with depression in pregnancy is that it can have a negative impact on obtaining and maintaining good prenatal health, particularly in the areas of nutrition, sleep habits, exercise and following care instructions from your physician or midwife. Self-medicating with substance abuse, including alcohol and cigarette smoking, also tends to be higher in pregnant women who report depression. There is also a higher risk of suicide.

Further, depression during pregnancy puts you at a higher risk of having postpartum depression. A large number of studies have demonstrated that prenatal depression is one of the strongest predictors of postpartum depression.

## How Do You Know If It Is Depression?

Many of the signs of depression mimic conditions associated with pregnancy. This can make it difficult to tell what is normal in pregnancy and what is depression. Depression and anxiety may also go undiagnosed because women often dismiss their feelings, or chalk them up to the temporary moodiness that often accompanies pregnancy.

This problem can lead to women not getting the necessary care and treatment they may need. There is also a tendency of friends and family to ignore the possibility of depression in pregnancy simply because of a misconception this is supposed to be the happiest time in a woman's life.

## Signs of Depression

*Below are some common symptoms of depression:*
- Problems concentrating
- Problems with sleeping; either sleeping too little or too much
- Having headaches, aches and pains, or stomach pains that won't go away
- Fatigue
- Changes in eating habits
- Losing interest or pleasure in activities you used to enjoy
- Feeling anxious
- Irritability
- Feelings of worthlessness and guilt
- Withdrawing from friends and family

## *What Should I Do If I'm Depressed?*

Don't be embarrassed about letting others know about your feelings and possible concerns about depression. Women can feel guilty about these feelings and may not disclose these feelings to others. It is just as important to take care of your emotional health as it is to take care of your physical health. In fact, it can affect your physical health and the health of your baby if you don't.

*According to recent studies, pregnant women with untreated depression are more likely to experience:*

- Preterm birth
- Spontaneous abortion
- Gestational hypertension or preeclampsia

Depression that is left untreated and continues after your birth has been found to pose serious risks for the quality of your mother-child interaction, interfering with the ability of you to bond with your baby and for your baby to form a secure attachment with you.

Treatment during pregnancy is very important. You can start by reaching out to your partner about how you are feeling. Talk with your physician or midwife about your concerns. Developing a strong support network of your family, friends, and your caregiver is extremely valuable. Surround yourself with supportive individuals. Talk to a professional; psychotherapy can be very beneficial, particularly since there are major changes happening during pregnancy. They can help address your concerns, recommend supportive measures and assist with treatment where appropriate.

Sometimes medications may be used for depression, as deemed necessary and appropriate, during pregnancy under the care of a practitioner who has experience with using antidepressants and other medications during the course of pregnancy and breastfeeding. There are still many unanswered questions about the safety and possible long term affects of their use. You should discuss the possible risks and benefits with your healthcare provider before considering or taking any antidepressant medications.

You need to understand that just as the food you eat affects your baby, so does your stress level and your emotional health. It is important that you minimize your stress, control your anxiety, and successfully deal with depression as much as possible during pregnancy. This will provide your baby the optimal environment in which to grow. Whether you are dealing with stressors during pregnancy, or maybe even have concerns about depression, through the use of these stress management techniques you can take the first and necessary steps in making your pregnancy a healthier and happier one.

# Nutrition for the First Trimester

## *The Pregnancy Diet Essentials*

Nutrition during pregnancy is serious business. What you eat plays a vital role in determining the health of that little one you are so anxiously awaiting. Contrary to common belief, it isn't how much you eat that's so important (in fact, a pregnant mom needs to increase her calorie intake only by 300 calories a day during the second and third trimester) – but what you eat.

Nutrition is the foundation of life. The quality of the first six months to twelve months of a baby's life is greatly affected by the mother's prenatal nutritional status and diet because the baby relies on the mother for all of its nutritional needs. If the nutrients are unavailable, the fetus will suffer. Nutrition impacts weight gain, birth weight, gestational age, congenital anomalies, nutritional status, and birth defects in the fetus, and predispose the child to resist or develop chronic diseases in later life.

**How much to gain:** If you enter pregnancy at a weight you are realistically happy with, you should gain between 25 and 35 pounds. Only two to four pounds of that happen during the first trimester, and the remainder is added at about a rate of three-quarters to one pound per week after that. For underweight moms, it is important to put on at least 28 to 40 pounds. If you've started with extra weight, try to add only 15 to 25 pounds.

By nature's design, when the nausea has calmed down, it's time to be more conscious of the healthy choices you make. It is important to remember that what you put in your mouth goes to your baby. If you don't put anything in your mouth that is healthy, your baby gets nothing healthy to eat.

**Weighty nutrients:** There are a few critical nutrients that play particularly important roles in fetal development. The increased demand on your system, plus the developing fetus, requires extra nutrients. Quality eating will help take care you get those needed nutrients, along with an appropriate supplement.

*Here is a list of pregnancy super foods that boost energy and provide needed nutrients for you and your baby:*

- Broccoli – a great source of beta carotene with vitamin C as well as sweet red peppers, strawberries, and oranges which help to keep you energized.
- Blueberries – contain protective antioxidants and stimulate the brain.
- Spinach – high in vitamins A and C as well as folate. It is also a good source of fiber.
- Oatmeal – a good source of complex carbohydrates providing your body with sustained energy and good fiber!
- Eggs – contain varying amounts of 13 vitamins plus many minerals. Egg protein is of such high quality that it is often used as the standard by which other protein is measured. Egg protein contains essential amino acids which are building blocks of protein which the body needs. An egg yolk is one of the few foods which contain vitamin D, the sunshine vitamin.
- Almonds – each ounce of almonds contains a good amount of the antioxidant vitamin E, six grams of protein and no cholesterol. Almonds are also an excellent source of magnesium and offer calcium, fiber, the B vitamin folate and phosphorus.

**Calories:** Despite that fact you don't need too many more, those extras that you do need are very important. Proper weight gain on your part is needed to make sure your newborn is delivered at a healthy weight. Add 200 to 300 calories per day during the second and third trimesters.

## 14 ACSS Mini-Meals for Growing Moms

When eating seems particularly difficult, try small amounts several times a day. This will help avoid experiencing nausea and heartburn.

Being creative with meals just doesn't happen when you don't feel good or don't have the time or energy, so here are some nutritious suggestions for healthy mini-meals we've tested as tried and true.

1. Half a whole wheat bagel with almond butter or tahini
2. Yogurt shake made with vanilla yogurt, banana and orange juice
3. Hard-boiled egg sliced onto a small salad

4.  Cup of chicken noodle soup and a square of whole grain cornbread
5.  Tofu salad on a whole wheat roll
6.  Small bran muffin (homemade or one you trust to be wholesome) and a tangerine
7.  Almond butter on cinnamon raisin toast
8.  Half a turkey sandwich in pita bread with sliced tomato and sprouts
9.  Cup of ginger tea and the other half of that whole wheat bagel.
10. Cold leftover chicken from last night with a few dried apricots
11. Bowl of whole grain cereal with soy milk or regular milk
12. Small bowl of low-fat granola topped with half a banana and a dollop of yogurt
13. Open-faced broiled low-fat cheese on whole wheat
14. Instant oatmeal with raisins

# Additional Pregnancy Diet Essentials

## *Protein*

**Why you need it:** Protein is essential to the very foundation of your baby's growth. Eating enough protein ensures that your little one, from the very beginning, is getting adequate food stores to support cell growth and blood production.

**Sources:** Look for lean cuts of meat (be wary of lunchmeat, unless it is heated to steaming), fish low in mercury, poultry, egg whites, beans, peanut butter, tofu, and nuts (almonds and cashews are especially protein-rich).

**Servings:** The March of Dimes suggests all pregnant women eat two to three servings of protein daily. That's equal to two ounces lean meat or poultry, two tablespoons nut butter, one-half cup beans (cooked or dried), or two eggs. (The US RDA for pregnant and lactating women is 60 to 80 grams of protein daily.)

## *Calcium*

**Why you need it:** To grow strong bones and teeth, and facilitate muscle contraction and nerve function, you and baby need plenty of calcium.

**Sources:** Milk, cheese, yogurt, spinach, sardines, and salmon (with bones).

**Servings:** You'll need two to three, one cup servings of milk or the equivalent (e.g., one ounce of cheese, one cup plain yogurt, or one cup of cottage cheese) every day. According to the US RDA for pregnant and lactating women, you should aim for 1,200 mg of calcium daily. (You can try taking supplements with meals throughout the day in 200 to 300 mg increments.)

## Fruits and Vegetables Rich in Vitamin C

**Why you need it:** The old adage, "an apple a day keeps the doctor away" holds true! This is especially so during pregnancy. Vitamin C helps you and your baby maintain healthy gums, teeth, and bones; it also assists with iron absorption.

**Sources:** Broccoli, cantaloupe, Brussels sprouts, honeydew melon, cauliflower, lemons, collard greens, oranges, green peppers, papaya, mustard greens, strawberries, potatoes, watermelon, tomatoes, spinach, and fortified fruit juices.

**Servings:** You should get one to two half cup servings of fruits and vegetables high in vitamin C each day. According to the American College of Obstetrics and Gynecology (ACOG), pregnant women require 85 mg of vitamin C daily.

## Fruits and Vegetables Rich in Beta-Carotene

**Why you need it:** Beta-carotene, which your body converts into vitamin A, is great for healthy skin, good eyesight, and growing bones.

**Sources:** Broccoli, apricots, cabbage, cantaloupe, carrots, nectarines, chard, papaya, kale, peaches, sweet potatoes, watermelon, spinach, pumpkin, and winter squash.

**Servings:** Two half cup servings from the above list of produce every other day, or one half cup serving daily. Your recommended daily allowance of beta-carotene or vitamin A during pregnancy is 770 mcg.

*Note:* Excessive vitamin A intake (>10,000 IU/day) may be associated with fetal malformations; speak with your healthcare provider to find out just how much you should take in your prenatal and how many beta-carotene rich foods you should incorporate into your diet.

# Carbohydrates

**Why you need it:** Going carb-free during pregnancy is not a good idea. You and your baby need those hearty grains! Carbs are important for helping you maintain daily energy production.

**Sources:** Breads, cereals, rice, potatoes, pasta, fruits, and vegetables.

**Servings:** The ACOG suggests you shoot for roughly six servings of carbs daily (one serving is roughly equal to one slice of bread, three-fourths cup dry cereal, or one-half cup cooked cereal or grains).

# Iron

**Why you need it:** Anemia can be a problem for pregnant women. Ensuring that you stay on top of your iron intake can help keep you from becoming anemic Your healthcare provider will check for anemia throughout your pregnancy. Eating iron-rich foods facilitates red blood cell production (too much can make you feel constipated, though, so be sure to speak with your healthcare provider about how much is best for you).

**Sources:** Lean red meat, spinach, and iron-fortified, whole grain breads and cereals are all good sources for iron. You may also take a prenatal vitamin with extra iron (speak with your health care provider first).

**Servings:** To get 30 mg, try for three to four ounces of meat, one cup beans, or one half cup tofu or boiled greens daily. If your health care provider recommends you take an iron supplement during pregnancy, ACOG suggests you look for one that offers 27 mg daily.

# Vitamin B6

**Why you need it:** In addition to helping your body manage stress, vitamin B6 also assists in red blood cell formation and effective use of protein, fat, and carbohydrates.

**Sources:** Whole grain cereals and pasta, brown rice, lean meats (such as pork), poultry, fish, avocados, beans, potatoes, corn, bananas, and nuts.

**Servings:** One potato, avocado, or banana; one cup of cereal, beans, or rice; three to four ounces of lean meat, fish, or poultry. The ACOG recommends all pregnant women get 1.9 mg of vitamin B6 daily.

## Vitamin B12

**Why you need it:** B12 is essential in the formation of red blood cells. It also helps maintain your and your baby's nervous system (which makes it wonderful for managing Mom-to-be-related stress)

**Sources:** Meat, fish, poultry, milk products, and fortified breakfast cereals

**Note:** If you're a vegetarian and don't eat any dairy products, it is important that you speak with your health care provider about regularly taking a B12 supplement.

**Servings:** You'll need to take in 2.6 mcg of B12 daily. That's about three to four ounces of meat, poultry, or fish; one cup yogurt, one ounce of cheese; or one cup dry cereal daily.

## Vitamin D

**Why you need it:** Both you and Baby need vitamin D to build and maintain healthy bones and teeth. Vitamin D also helps the body's absorption of calcium.

**Sources:** Only a few foods, like egg yolks, fatty fish, and cod liver oil, naturally contain vitamin D. It is often added to fortify milk, dairy products, breads and cereals, too. Sunlight is another good source of vitamin D.

**Servings:** In addition to the recommended daily allowance for dairy, breads, and cereals, you can ensure you're getting enough vitamin D by adding one teaspoon (15 mL) of cod liver oil to your daily diet. You'll need 5 mcg of vitamin D daily during pregnancy. Or be outside for 25 minutes each day and enjoy sun on your face and hands. These simple tricks can help your body synthesize a sufficient amount of vitamin D.

## Folic Acid

**Why you need it:** The March of Dimes recommends that all women trying to conceive or who are pregnant take folic acid to lessen the possibility of their babies developing birth defects. Folic acid, a B vitamin, also helps blood and protein production and encourages effective enzyme function.

**Sources:** Shop for green, leafy vegetables, dark yellow fruits and vegetables, beans, peas, and nuts.

**Servings:** Two cups fresh leafy greens (or one cup boiled greens); one cup beans, peas, or nuts; and one orange, tomato, or carrot. Healthcare providers also recommend that all pregnant women, as well as those trying to conceive, take a supplement containing 400 mcg of folic acid.

## Healthy Fats

**Why you need it:** Believe it or not, fat should be a part of your pregnancy diet. But make sure it is the right kind of fat: avoid trans fats and look for omega-3s and unsaturated fats.

**Sources:** Meat, fish, whole milk dairy products, nuts, peanut butter, avocado, olive and canola oils.

**Servings:** Two servings of fatty fish per week; salmon is a good choice during pregnancy. Be sure to limit fat intake to 30% or less of your total daily calorie intake. (If you are eating about 2,000 calories a day, this would be 65 grams of fat or less.)

## Water

**Why you need it:** Staying hydrated during pregnancy is essential. Water provides your body with a path for transporting nutrients for you and your growing baby. Water feeds yours and Baby's cells, balances your bodies' acids and salts, and contributes to the cushioning of your cells and organs. Drinking plenty of water also ensures that your baby will have a good level of fluid in which to grow and develop in your womb.

**Sources:** Although some foods are rich in water (watermelon, for example), drinking water is your best bet.

**Servings:** You'll need to drink eight to twelve, eight-ounce glasses of water every day.

# Exercise in the First Trimester

Attitudes and beliefs about prenatal exercise have drastically changed over the past twenty years. We no longer look at pregnancy as a time to sit and watch TV and each chocolate. These days, moms can actually maintain and improve their fitness levels while pregnant. And exercise provides many numerous benefits besides a healthy *weight gain!*

*Some of the benefits of exercise include:*
- Less aches and pains
- Eliminates or reduces pregnancy-related discomforts
- Helps prevent gestational diabetes
- Improves calcium absorption, preventing hypertension, preeclampsia, and future osteoporosis
- Relieves tension, stress, and possible depression
- Increases your general strength
- Reduces the strain on your upper back
- Reduces the strain and pressure on your sciatic nerve
- Prevents "rounded shoulders"
- Increases energy, particularly in the last trimester
- Improves your immunity
- Helps minimizes stretch marks – *we moms love this one!!!*
- Helps minimize postpartum blues and depression
- Allows faster recovery from pregnancy, labor and birth
- Helps you get back into shape quicker

*Exercise has also been shown to:*
- Decrease the need for pain relief during labor
- Decrease the incidence of maternal exhaustion – or prevent Mom from getting to the point where she cannot tolerate labor anymore
- May help decrease the need for a c-section

## *Common Complaints from Moms in the First Trimester:*

**I'm tired.** Naps are a necessary element of your first trimester exercise program.

**My breasts are sore.** Make sure you're wearing great-fitting sports bras, and maybe it's time to try something new!

**I constantly need to use the ladies room.** You have elevated levels of progesterone, so you'll need more frequent restroom breaks.

**I'm nauseous.** Your body has elevated estrogen and HCG levels. This should get better in the second and third trimesters. In the meantime, carry a small snack to the gym and check out our section on nausea for more tips.

**I have heartburn.** Again, with your elevated progesterone levels, this may or may not get better so a good tip is to keep antacids in your gym bag!

## *Exercise Modifications*

**Keep your heart rate under 140 beats per minute!** Actually follow the talk test, i.e. if you can talk to your neighbor you are ok.

**Be careful to not overheat.** Keep ice water on hand and go slower if you need to.

You should be able maintain your current fitness program, but be sure to discuss it with your healthcare provider.

## *Physiological Changes*

These are changes you're going to see in your body that can affect exercise and begin happening from day one.

**Lungs and Breathing:** In pregnancy the respiratory rate is naturally increased because more oxygenated blood is needed for both Mom and Baby. This may cause Mom to feel breathlessness, especially during a workout. Use the talk test method: if can you talk to your neighbor while exercising, you are probably at a good workout intensity.

**Musculoskeletal:** Because of your growing uterus, the lower back develops more curvature and the center of gravity for your body shifts. This can cause changes in your sense of balance and requires adjustments in posture to prevent injury.

The joints also undergo changes during pregnancy. Your body releases a hormone called relaxin, which loosens up the joints of the pelvis to make room for the birth of your child. Because all of the joints in the body are more lax, there is a greater chance of spraining or straining muscles and joints during pregnancy and increase the chance of falling.

**Metabolism:** During pregnancy your body uses carbohydrates more quickly. Exercise also increases the metabolism of carbohydrates. These two factors can lead to low blood sugar reactions during exercise. Increasing caloric intake to shift your carbohydrate balance is very important. Always carry extra food to the gym with you.

**Cardiovascular:** Your body increases its blood volume by 50% in pregnancy. In addition, your heart rate increases by about 15 beats per minute. This allows nutrients and oxygen to be transported to the fetus more efficiently. This increase in blood volume is also partly responsible for the swelling we endure in our ankles, hands, and feet. With the growth of your uterus, the flow of blood in your body can be disrupted and lightheadedness can occur. Be aware of these physiological changes so you can adapt accordingly.

**Elevated Body Temperature:** Exercise causes an increase in core body temperature, and so it is important to stay cool while exercising. Avoid exercising outside during the summer months. Join a gym and take classes in air-conditioned studios. Not only will the heat make you feel nauseated but the baby has no way of cooling him/herself down, so Mom needs to make sure she stays cool. If you do feel overheated seek shade, grab some cool water and reduce the level of activity you are doing. When you feel better you can begin again. And ALWAYS make sure you drink plenty of water.

## *Complications of Pregnancy that May Affect Exercise*

**Anemia (or a low blood count):** Results in lower oxygen carrying capacity of your blood. This has a big impact on endurance and may result in a marked decrease in your exercise capability because of breathlessness, dizziness and fatigue. Women with anemia who want to continue their exercise program should eat an iron-rich diet, take extra vitamin C with meals to increase iron absorption and should take iron supplements if prescribed by their healthcare provider. Be sure to take your iron supplement separate from your prenatal vitamin for better absorption.

**Contractions:** Some women experience preterm contractions throughout their pregnancy. While preterm contractions do not always lead to preterm birth, they do increase a woman's risk of preterm labor significantly. If you have frequent contractions during your pregnancy, strenuous exercise may lead to a higher rate of contractions. Exercise programs should be adjusted to include more non-weight bearing exercise like yoga, stretching and swimming rather than speed walking or jogging.

**Lower Back Pain or Sciatica:** Many women have episodes of lower back pain or leg pain during pregnancy because of weight changes and changes in body posture. Weight-bearing exercise can increase pain levels and further stress the joints. Again, non-weight bearing exercise may help with these symptoms. Swimming is particularly helpful.

**Toxemia/Pre-eclampsia/High Blood Pressure:** Women who develop high blood pressure in pregnancy should stop their exercise program. Toxemia, pre-eclampsia or pregnancy induced hypertension that develops during pregnancy, is thought to involve a severe problem with the blood vessels throughout the body. Exercise can worsen this condition and should be discontinued.

**Placenta Previa/Vaginal Bleeding:** Placenta Previa is a condition where the placenta grows low in the uterus and actually covers the opening to the cervix. It can cause severe bleeding during pregnancy. Any woman with placenta previa or with vaginal bleeding of an unknown cause should not participate in an exercise program.

**Preterm Labor or History or Preterm Labor:** Women who have delivered a baby before 36 weeks of pregnancy should be very cautious in participating in an exercise program during the second and third trimesters of pregnancy. Stretching, yoga and walking are preferred forms of exercise, while weight-bearing exercise should be avoided. Also, women with preterm contractions should avoid exercise that increases uterine contractions, whether painful or painless.

**Intrauterine Growth Restriction (IUGR):** Poor growth of the baby. Your healthcare provider diagnoses IUGR by measuring the growth of your uterus and by checking a fetal sonogram. If your baby has IUGR, it may mean that the baby is not getting an adequate oxygen supply from the placenta. There are many causes of IUGR including smoking, drug use, infections and poor blood flow to the placenta. Because exercise shifts blood flow away from the placenta, a baby that is not growing well will not tolerate exercise by its mom.

**Twin Pregnancy:** Women who are pregnant with more than one fetus have a higher risk of complications during pregnancy including preterm labor. Exercise should be limited to non-weight bearing and should focus on toning and stretching. Talk to your healthcare provider about limitations.

**Heart Disease:** Exercise increases the strain on the heart, as does pregnancy because of increased blood volume. Women with heart problems should exercise only under the supervision of their cardiologist and healthcare provider.

---

### Reasons to Stop Exercising

Stop exercising and tell your healthcare provider if you experience any of the following:

- Blood or fluid coming from your vagina
- Sudden or severe abdominal or vaginal pain
- Contractions that go on for 30 minutes after you stop exercising
- Chest pain
- Shortness of breath
- Headache that is severe or won't go away
- Dizziness
- Dim or blurry vision

---

## Designing a Prenatal Exercise Plan

- Ask your healthcare provider if it is ok! If you have been working out prior to pregnancy and are having a healthy pregnancy you should have no problems continuing.
- Let any instructors/trainers/friends you workout with know you are expecting, as they can help provide useful guidelines and tips.

- Not sure where to begin? Seek the advice of a prenatal certified personal trainer or download one of the ACSS templates online at www.9monthsin9monthsout.com.
- Listen to your body. If it says stop or slow down, listen, otherwise you run the risk of throwing up on the treadmill. (Yes, Corry did this. Needless to say, very embarrassing, especially when no one knows you are pregnant yet!)
- Wear comfortable workout clothes and shoes.
- Drink lots of water before, during and after your workout.
- Not a yoga or Pilates fan? Try a class. You may really enjoy it during pregnancy!
- Visit our website for more ACSS tips, exercises, and recommended classes!

The best part of exercise when you are pregnant... it is fulfilling and helps build your endurance and strength, which will help you deal with your laboring and birth process.

# Relaxation & Stress Management for the First Trimester

Stress impacts every aspect of our lives. There are external stressors and internal stressors and honestly, stress is all in how we react to a given situation. People don't stress us out. We let them stress us out. That guy who cut you off in traffic? He can't hear you. You can't change the fact that he cut you off. Ask yourself this question: Is this something I can change? If yes, then change it. If no, then let it go. (And if yes, and you're just not ready to change it, then that's acceptable too, just stop beating yourself up over it.)

A few ways to manage and reduce stress, other than that already mentioned (exercise, massage, and nutrition), is to key in and listen to ourselves and our babies during the pregnancy, including:

**Breathing Exercises** – This provides numerous benefits for the body, including oxygenating the blood, which 'wakes up' the brain, relaxing muscles and quieting the mind. Breathing exercises work quickly so you can de-stress in a matter of a few short breaths. Practice by sitting up straight in your chair. When breathing in, pull your navel to your spine, and fill your lungs upward, thus In and Up. When breathing out, reverse it, breathing Out and Down. This is a reverse breathing pattern traditionally taught in Qi Gong and Tai Chi. It requires a unique focus to keep the breath cycle going. Try this for three deep breaths to start, and use the technique whenever you're feeling stressed.

**Meditation** – Taking your breathing exercises one step further, when you meditate, your brain enters an area of functioning that's similar to sleep, but carries some added benefits including the release of certain hormones that promote health. Also, the mental focus on nothingness keeps your mind from working overtime which could increase your stress level.

**Guided Imagery** – It takes slightly more time to practice guided imagery, but this is a great way to leave your stress behind for a while and relax your body. Some find it easier to practice guided imagery than meditation, as lots of us find it more doable to focus on 'something' than on 'nothing.' You can play natural sounds in the background as you practice to promote a more immersive experience.

**Visualizations** – Building on guided imagery, you can also visualize yourself achieving goals like becoming healthier and more relaxed, doing well at tasks, and handling conflict in better ways. Also, imagining yourself doing well on tasks you're trying to master actually functions like physical practice, so you can improve your performance through visualizations as well!

**Self-hypnosis** – Self-hypnosis incorporates some of the features of guided imagery and visualizations, with the added benefit of enabling you to communicate directly with your subconscious mind to enhance your abilities. It can help you give up bad habits more easily, feel less pain, develop healthier habits more effectively, and even find answers to questions that may not be clear to your waking mind! It takes some practice and training, but is well worth it. Learn more about using hypnosis to manage stress in your life.

**Progressive Muscle Relaxation** – By tensing and relaxing all the muscle groups in your body, you can relieve tension and feel much more relaxed in minutes, with no special training or equipment. Start by tensing all the muscles in your face, holding a tight grimace ten seconds, then completely relaxing for ten seconds. Repeat this with your neck, followed by your shoulders, etc. You can do this anywhere, and as you practice, you will find you can relax more quickly and easily, reducing tension as quickly as it starts!

**Music** – Music therapy has shown numerous health benefits for people with mild to severe conditions ranging from stress to cancer. When dealing with stress, the right music can actually lower your blood pressure, relax your body and calm your mind.

Rather than using just one of the techniques mentioned above, it is best to combine a few aspects, giving yourself and your baby the chance to de-stress and relax during pregnancy and birth.

For the first trimester, start to build yourself a nightly routine, one that you can perhaps carry over to sharing with your little one when he/she arrives. Give yourself a chance to unwind from the day. With soft music, or after a warm bath or shower, practice your breathing techniques or even use a premade hypnosis CD to help you focus on good thoughts and actions for your pregnancy.

## Example Relaxation Technique

You can find a copy of this Guided Relaxation on the Nine Months In Nine Months Out web site www.9monthsin9monthsout.com. Please use the code: GR8RLX to download a free MP3.

Find a comfortable spot. Take a few deep breaths in and up, out and down. Allow yourself to unwind from the day and enjoy this relaxation (visualization) technique.

*Imagine you are in the most relaxing space you know. It can be a warm summer's day on the beach, or a cool autumn afternoon near a mountain lake. Wherever your most relaxing space is, go there. And as you lie motionless, imagine a warm white light just above your head. This white light is the most relaxing light you can imagine.*

*Allow the warmth of the light to flow down, over your forehead, feeling all little frown lines, all the little worry lines, simply melt away.*

*Letting the warmth flow down over your eyes, your eyelids become warm and heavy, so heavy they don't even seem to want to open. They may flutter a little bit, but that's okay, just feel how heavy they are. Feel the relaxation spread down over your face, let all the muscles in your face unwind and relax. Allow the warmth flow over your lips, and into your jaw. Feel the warmth flow into your ears and around the back of your head. Feel your whole head grow warm and relaxed.*

*The relaxation flows down the back of your neck now all the way through to your throat, feeling any blocks release and let go. Allow the relaxation to spread down into your shoulders, feeling them drop a little. Feel the warmth spread into your arms, down around your elbows, and into your forearms. Allow the relaxation to wind around your wrists, flowing deep into your hands so that each and every finger relaxes more and more, more and more, as you go deeper and deeper into relaxation.*

*Now, allow the warmth to come back up to your throat and flow down into your chest. Feel your heart relax. Feel your lungs relax. Let the relaxation flow all the way through to your back. Feel your shoulder blades release and unwind. Feel the warm white light flow all the way down your spine and around to your sides. Allow the relaxation to flow deep into your stomach, feeling all the muscles, all the organs within your stomach release and let go. Feel the warmth flow down into your hips, allowing your hips to release and unwind.*

*Allow the warmth to flow down into the fronts of your thighs and all the way through to the backs. Down into the hollows of your knees, around to the knee itself. Feel the warmth flow down into your shins, all the way through to your calves. Feel the warmth flow down into your ankles and deep into the foot itself. Feel each and every toe relax more and more, more and more, as you go deeper and deeper into relaxation.*

*Take a deep breath in and up, out and down. Allow your whole body to feel warm, safe and secure. Nice and relaxed. Just allow yourself to go deeper and deeper and even deeper into relaxation.*

*Now, imagine yourself standing, and at the base of your feet is a beautiful stone stairway that leads downward into a very safe valley of relaxation. This staircase will lead you to a profound state of deep, deep relaxation. Going down these stairs now, count backwards from ten to zero, each number will take you even deeper, and deeper, and even deeper into your relaxed state.*

*Ten. Taking that first step down now.*

*Nine, deeper and deeper.*

*Eight, way down now.*

*Seven, deeper... and deeper.*

*Six... deeper, feeling very relaxed now....*

*Five... deeper and deeper.*

*Four... you are going into a deep state of relaxation now.*

*Three, going deeper....*

*Two, relaxed even more, feeling very calm.*

*One. At the next number, you will enter this beautiful place of peace and tranquility called deep, deep relaxation. More relaxed and peaceful than you've ever known yourself to be.*

*And, zero.*

*Now, in a moment, count from five to one. When you reach the count of one, your legs are going to be soooo relaxed, so heavy, that you will not be able to lift them.*

*Five – getting heavier and heavier now.*

*Four – more and more relaxed as you imagine the relaxation flowing through all the muscles in your legs.*

*Three – so deeply relaxed now as you imagine that relaxation flowing deep down into your bones.*

*Two – so relaxed, too relaxed to even move as you go from two…
down to… one. Now, try to lift your legs and find with a bit of
amusement that you cannot. They are just too heavy.*

*That's right, don't even try any more, they are just too relaxed.*

*Slowly begin to count backwards from five to one. Allow your
eyes to become 100 times heavier than your legs just were. So heavy,
they will not be able to open, no matter how much you try.*

*Five – feel the relaxation flowing around your eyes now.*

*Four – the relaxation crosses the bridge of your nose and flows
thru the temples.*

*Three – feel the relaxation now flowing deep down into your
eyes, all the way thru your head.*

*Two – so relaxed, too relaxed to open your eyes as you go from
two down to one. So relaxed now, your eyes will not be able to open,
but try. Try to open your eyes only when you are certain that you
cannot.*

*That's right, don't even try anymore, they are just too heavy.*

*Very good. That's right. Just continuing to go deeper and deeper,
relaxing. As you continue to listen to the sound of the music, simply
allow your body to relax to sleep. A deep, warm, comfortable,
healing sleep. Letting the rest and relaxation flow from you to baby.
Simply… drifting… relaxing… sleeping deeply now.*

## Massage in the First Trimester

The main role of massage in the first trimester is to improve healthy circulation
and, in general, relaxation. Massage has been shown to decrease norepinephrine
and cortical hormones ("stress hormones") and also to boost levels of dopamine
and serotonin (low levels of these hormones are associated with depression). It is a

known fact that one of the causes of premature birth is stress. Massage can very effectively help to lower stress levels.

You will find publications that recommend not getting massages in the first trimester. The claim is that massage can cause a miscarriage. While there is no scientific data to support the theory that pressure to specific areas on the body can stimulate labor, there are many who believe caution to be wise. The points that have been most commonly pointed out as areas to avoid receiving vigorous massage are the areas around the inner side of the ankle, below the inner knee area and the soft tissue between the thumb and forefinger. This does not mean that you cannot get a foot rub or if you happen to find yourself absently rubbing at those areas that there is cause for alarm. Even the most extreme of these publications specify "vigorous, specific, pinpointed pressure."

During the first trimester, massage is very much the same as before pregnancy. There is not yet a reason to need any special positioning (unless there are issues with heartburn) or to change any regular routines. You should, however, inform your massage therapist of the pregnancy and work in the common endangerment sights. Being an educated mom and taking the initiative to know what you're comfortable with is always recommended. Ask your massage therapist about his or her experience with prenatal massage and speak up if the massage is too intense in areas you are not comfortable with.

Many women experience headaches in the first few months of pregnancy, even those whom have never experienced problems with headaches in the past. There are many theories as to why this is but no definitive answers. It is generally found that relaxation massage is a good way to find relief from these unexplained headaches. Another method is hot cold hydrotherapy.

---

**Massage Cautions**

*High-risk disorders (talk with your healthcare provider first)*

- DVT (deep vein thrombosis)
- High blood pressure
- Preeclampsia

*Massage techniques not to use during pregnancy*

- Heat packs or heating pads around abdomen and flanks
- Breast massage
- Very intense massage of any sort

*Massage oils, skin care products and aromatherapies to avoid include:*

- Any anti-wrinkle cream containing Retin-A
- Essential oils of basil, cedar wood, cinnamon, clary sage (during labor), clove, cypress (after 5 months), fennel, geranium (avoid in early pregnancy), hyssop, jasmine (during labor), juniper, lemongrass, myrrh, parsley, and pennyroyal. There is conflicting advice about which oils are safe and which are not. When in doubt, consult with your local aromatherapist.

---

## Finding a Massage Therapist

Referrals are always best. Ask your friends or ask for recommendations from your doctor, midwife, hospital or your regular massage therapist if they don't do prenatal massage themselves. You can also check your local spas and chiropractic offices.

*Questions to ask a prospective massage therapist include:*
- How much prenatal massage training do you have?
- How much experience do you have in performing prenatal massage?
- How long have you been doing massage therapy?

- How long have you been doing prenatal massage?
- How will you handle positioning me as I progress through my pregnancy?
- Ask the therapist to discuss the difference between traditional massage and prenatal massage with you.

It may feel overwhelming deciding what type of massage and which therapist is best for you. There are many different modalities or styles of massage out there. Typically, it is best to go with someone who specializes specifically in prenatal massage or has extensive experience and training in prenatal massage as well as other techniques. The most common types are the following: Swedish Massage, Relaxation Massage, Full Body Massage and Circulation Massage; they all refer to the basic full body, relaxation massage.

## *Some Common Massage Modalities*

**Swedish Full Body Relaxation** – Every therapist has their own style but the intention is to ease tension in muscles, improve circulation and overall relaxation. Long, smooth strokes flowing toward the heart are used along with other types of kneading, rolling and broadening strokes to achieve overall relaxation.

**Deep Tissue Massage** – A more intense technique intended to address specific tensions and pains. Similar strokes as in a Swedish massage are used to warm and prepare an area, the pressure gets progressively firmer and the use of static pressure is often applied to break up knotted up areas in the muscles. *You may want to use this modality sparingly as the pregnancy progresses.*

**Shiatsu** – Developed in Japan, Shiatsu is a technique using traditional acupuncture points with the intension of unblocking the flow of energy through the body. Pressure is applied using fingers, thumbs, palm, elbow or knee to specific points correlating with the lines thought to be energy pathways through the body called Meridians. This treatment brings about a sense of relaxation and stimulates blood and lymphatic flow.

**Reflexology** – A technique based on an ancient Chinese therapy, this is a method using manipulation of specific areas in the hands, feet or ears that reflexively correspond to other parts of the body. Similar to the principles behind acupressure and acupuncture, Reflexology is meant to interact with the body's energy flow to aid in self-healing and maintain balance in physical function. It is very important that a therapist offering Reflexology to pregnant women be very knowledgeable and experienced in both Prenatal massage and Reflexology as there are pressure points in the hands and feet which are believed to be unsafe to work on during pregnancy.

**Aromatherapy** – This is the use of essential oils (extracted from herbs, flowers, woods, resins and roots) in body and skin care. Aromatherapy has been used for thousands of years as an aid in relaxation and healing. In an aromatherapy massage the essential oils can be used either in the massage oil or in a diffuser to scent the air in the room.

# Conclusion

Congratulations! You've made it through the first third of your pregnancy. Most moms say the second trimester is the best part of pregnancy because you're less nauseous, and more energetic.

# Second Trimester

Your body is changing. Morning sickness has finally started to pass. Your belly is beginning to grow. This is the most stable part of your pregnancy. Your clothes may start getting tight, or not fitting at all. Delight in it all!

## Second Trimester Development

| Timeframe | Development |
|---|---|
| *Twelve to Fifteen Weeks* | If you could see inside the uterus, the sex of the baby would be easy to identify. |
| | The ears, arms, hands, fingers, legs, feet and toes are formed. |
| | The neck is well shaped and can support the head. |
| | Reflex movements allow your baby's elbows to bend, legs to kick and fingers to form a fist. |
| | Your baby's vocal cords are formed. |
| | Blood is now traveling through the umbilical cord to the baby and will continue to do so until the cord is cut at delivery. |
| | The face is looking more and more human each day as the eyes begin to move closer together instead of being on the sides of the head and the ears move to a normal position. |
| | The intestines move farther into the baby's body; the liver begins to produce insulin. |
| | Your baby begins to practice inhaling and exhaling movements. |
| | Your baby will weigh about ¼ pound and will be about 2 ¼ inches long. |
| *Sixteen to Nineteen Weeks* | All of the organs have developed. |
| | Beneath the gums, teeth are forming. |
| | Fine hair begins to grow all over the body; this downy hair is called lanugo. |
| | Your baby's heart is pumping about 25 quarts of blood each day. |

| | |
|---|---|
| | Fingernails and toenails begin to form, and the baby sucks and swallows.<br><br>The legs are now longer than the arms.<br><br>Pads are forming on the fingertips and toes, and the eyes are looking forward rather than out the sides of the head.<br><br>Meconium, the baby's first bowel movement, is accumulating within the bowel.<br><br>About one cup of amniotic fluid surrounds your baby.<br><br>The baby's kidneys now circulate the fluid swallowed by the baby back into the amniotic sac.<br><br>The baby actively kicks its legs and moves its arms, but not with enough strength for you to be able to feel much movement.<br><br>It is possible, however, that you will start to feel a slight "flutter" type of movement when you are still.<br><br>By the end of the fourth month the baby is 3-4 inches long and weighs 5-6 ounces.<br><br>The uterus is about four inches in diameter and the mother's tummy may show a slight bulge. |
| *Twenty to Twenty Seven Weeks* | This continues to be a period of rapid growth.<br><br>Your baby is almost fully formed and looks like a miniature human. However, because the lungs are not well developed and the baby is still very small, he/she cannot usually live outside the uterus at this stage without highly specialized care.<br><br>Your baby's skin is wrinkled and red.<br><br>It is covered with lanugo (fine soft hair) and vernix (a substance consisting of oil, sloughed skin cells and lanugo).<br><br>Real hair and toenails are beginning to grow.<br><br>Your baby's brain is developing rapidly.<br><br>Fatty sheaths which transport impulses along nerves are forming.<br><br>A special type of fat (brown fat) that keeps your baby warm at birth is forming.<br><br>Baby girls will develop eggs in their ovaries during this time.<br><br>The baby's bones are becoming solid.<br><br>By the end of the sixth month, your baby will be around 11 to 14 inches long and will weigh about 1 to 1 ½ pounds. |

Table 4. Developing in the Second Trimester.

# Medical Considerations

As you progress through your second trimester, your healthcare provider will discuss the recommended tests for you and your baby that will be done. You will have a test called a one-hour glucose challenge test that is a screening test for Gestational Diabetes. You will also have your complete blood count (CBC) checked at this time.

Gestational diabetes is a condition that causes high levels of glucose in the blood. Glucose is a sugar that is the body's main source of fuel. Health problems can arise when the glucose levels are too high or not well controlled. Gestational diabetes is of special concern during pregnancy. It occurs when there is a problem with the way your body makes or uses insulin. Insulin is a hormone that converts the glucose in food into energy. When the body doesn't make enough insulin, or when your body is not using insulin properly, the level of glucose in the blood becomes too high. This is called hyperglycemia (high sugar levels in the blood). Because gestational diabetes can occur even when no risk factors of symptoms are present, all moms are tested between 25-28 weeks of pregnancy. Gestational diabetes does resolve after your baby is born. More than half of women who have gestational diabetes are at a higher risk of developing diabetes later in life. It's important to let your healthcare provider know if you have had gestational diabetes with a previous pregnancy or if you have a strong family history of diabetes.

The test for gestational diabetes is safe and simple.

- On the morning of your test, do not have any concentrated sweets for breakfast. Avoid fruit juices, sugary cereals, syrups, jellies, etc. Watch your carbohydrate intake! When you arrive for your appointment, let the receptionist know that you need to drink your glucola. This is a sugar drink (50 grams of sugar) that will be given to you. You should drink the glucola over a five minute period.
- For the next hour, do not have anything to eat or drink. Do not chew any gum or smoke (which you shouldn't be doing anyway!).
- At the end of the hour, your blood is drawn.
- You will be notified if your blood level is 135 or greater. Normal results will be reviewed at your next appointment.

- High levels (greater than 135) do not mean that you have gestational diabetes. A high value means that you need further testing and you will be scheduled for a three hour glucose tolerance test (3hr GTT) which is the diagnostic test for gestational diabetes.
- If your 3 hour test values are abnormal, you are diagnosed with gestational diabetes and will need diabetic education regarding diet, testing your blood sugars and follow-up. Your healthcare provider will provide you with the proper guidance needed.

# Nutrition in Your Second Trimester

Whew, most of you have made it through the phase where everything you look at or smell makes you want to throw up, but this is not a license to eat everything in sight. The second trimester is when healthcare professionals recommend increasing your daily calories by 200-300 per day. However, what you eat is just as important as adding those calories in. Why? You want to make a habit of choosing a variety of healthy foods for your growing baby.

*A healthy and balanced daily diet for Mom includes:*
- 3-5 servings of fresh fruits and vegetables. One of these servings needs to be a dark orange vegetable, and two should be of leafy, dark green vegetables. This will provide a variety of nutrients for both Mom and Baby.
- 2 servings of extra-lean meats, chicken, fish, or cooked peas or beans.
- At least 8 glasses of water.
- 6 servings of grains.
- 3 servings of non-fat or low-fat milk products.

Below are some of the important dietary tips for you to make your second trimester pregnancy diet healthy and well-balanced. If you have questions about health and nutrition during the second trimester, or at any other point during pregnancy, your healthcare provider will point you in the right direction, and help you map out a healthy eating plan.

**Limit Your Sugar** - Try to limit your excess sugar consumption, which can lead to unnecessary additional weight gain. Excess weight gain increases your odds for developing gestational diabetes, macrosomia and risk for a cesarean section. Look for "no sugar added" options and avoid adding sugar in your juices or other beverages.

**Limit Certain Foods** - It's best to avoid certain types of fish that may contain high levels of mercury. Uncooked meats, raw eggs, soft cheeses (unpasteurized dairy) and certain seafood can put you at a greater risk for listeria and salmonella. Even smoked seafood, if it is refrigerated, can increase the risk of listeria. Deli meats and hot dogs are not recommended for these reasons as well.

**Get Enough Iron** - It is important to continue taking your prenatal vitamin throughout pregnancy and postpartum, especially if nursing. Your prenatal vitamin contains the key mineral iron. Iron is important for the production of red blood cells for both Mom and Baby. The second trimester is when Mom's blood volume doubles in order to support the pregnancy. Iron is part of hemoglobin, which carries oxygen and other nutrients to the baby, and takes waste products out of the baby's system. Sometimes it's not possible to get enough iron to meet your body's needs during pregnancy through food and your prenatal vitamin alone; an iron supplement may be prescribed. Be sure to take them!

If the iron supplement irritates your stomach, tell your healthcare provider. There are many different types of iron supplements available and changing brands may help. Try taking iron supplements in the evening if you have morning sickness, and with food to help reduce stomach irritation. Also, be sure to drink plenty of fluids because iron supplements may cause constipation. Iron deficiency anemia can be harmful to both you and your baby. You are your baby's only source of oxygen, and iron carries oxygen through the blood. Your baby's organs, including his/her brain, are growing rapidly during the second trimester, so be sure to eat a well-balanced diet.

**Dairy Products** - Dairy products like milk, yogurt, cheese, cottage cheese, etc. are essential during the second trimester. Try to consume one glass of milk daily but make sure that you drink 2%, 1% or skim milk. Avoid vitamin D or whole milk. The only difference between these types of milk listed is the fat content. Dairy products are a rich source of calcium and are essential for the healthy growth of your child. So enjoy dairy products while you are pregnant. You need all the calcium you can get and so does your baby!

**Fresh Vegetables and Fruits** - Fresh vegetables and fruits are an important part of your second trimester diet. Make sure that you include 3-5 servings of fresh fruits and vegetables.

**Fiber Rich Diet** - During the second trimester constipation is very common and it can be incredibly uncomfortable. A diet rich in fiber will help.

**High Fat or Greasy** - Try to cut down on all junk and fat-filled food. While a big, greasy cheeseburger from your favorite fast food joint might be a daily pregnancy craving, it is not one that you should give into.

Cravings will come and go. Choose a wide variety of foods in your daily diet, take your prenatal vitamin and drink plenty of fresh water. Your body will thank you after pregnancy when it has less weight to lose than if you had indulged in those empty calories.

# Exercise in the Second Trimester

During the second trimester of pregnancy, your body's changes tend to be less severe, in regards to exercising (morning sickness, sore breasts) than in the first trimester of pregnancy. And they tend to be less severe than the bodily changes that occur during the third trimester of pregnancy. One of the biggest second trimester body changes, and the one that most often makes pregnant women very excited, is the fact that sometime between 18 and 22 weeks of pregnancy, or about halfway through the second trimester of pregnancy, you will be able to feel your baby move! Also during the second trimester your body will begin to gain weight more steadily. On the average, a pregnant woman will gain around one half to one pound each week. Both of these changes require small changes in your exercise routine to keep both Mom and Baby safe.

*Important Second Trimester Exercise Guidelines include:*
- Avoid exercises that require you to lie on your back for 60 seconds or longer, as the baby's increased weight can place pressure on your inferior vena cava (large blood vessel that returns blood to the mom's heart), which can decrease oxygen to both you and your baby. If you feel faint while on your back, roll over on your side to reestablish blood flow.

- Be careful of overheating, which can raise the heart rate of both you and your baby. A good way to watch for overheating is by using a heart rate monitor and keeping your heart rate under 140bpm.
- Sometime during this trimester, you will want to shop for a new sports bra, because your existing one is probably getting too tight.
- If you feel unbalanced during these weeks, consider discontinuing any activity that can throw you off balance, such as tennis, skating, trail biking, and hiking in the woods. Replace your old routine with new favorites like swimming, water aerobics, or a stationary bike, which don't require as much balance.
- Because your baby is growing and becoming more vulnerable in this trimester, if you fall or are hit in the abdomen, the baby may be harmed. Enjoy trying different exercises that aren't contact sports or risk fall or injury. Due to your expanding abdomen, you may find a recumbent bike more comfortable than a traditional stationary bike.
- If you're doing step aerobics, make sure that your step is no higher than four inches off the ground to help maintain a steady, stable balance.
- If you're rowing, you may find that this super-intense sport is too fatiguing for the rest of your pregnancy. Pay careful attention to how you're feeling and how well you and your baby are gaining weight.
- If you're weightlifting, don't overwork your thigh muscles; machines that work the thighs also tend to place stress on the ligaments around the pelvis and cause discomfort.
- If you're doing yoga, now's the time to stop doing back bends, any moves that have you lying on your stomach or back, jumps, and inverted poses.
- Focus on abdominals, lower back and Kegels.

---

### Don't Overstretch

Be careful during this trimester (and the next, and for about five months after you deliver) not to overstretch or make sudden moves. While you're pregnant, a hormone called relaxin prepares you for childbirth by relaxing all your ligaments and joints. This means that you may be at risk of injuring yourself because your joints and ligaments won't stop you from overextending yourself as well as they did when you weren't pregnant.

---

## *Abdominal Training*

Many women fear abdominal training during pregnancy, but there are exercises that are safe and effective during pregnancy. The benefits of strong and flexible abdominals in pregnancy include: minimizing backaches, promotion of good posture, and providing some support for the growing uterus.

The abdominals are made up of several different muscles.

**Transverse abdominis muscle** is the deepest support layer and wraps horizontally around the mid-section. It is the transverse that stretches the most during pregnancy yet still acts as a girdle.

**Rectus abdominis** or the Six-Pack muscle is the muscle that most people associate as the "abs." This muscle runs vertically from the pelvis to the ribs and is divided into two halves, whose primary function is to bend the spine forward. Diastasis recti or the separation of the abdominals during pregnancy is a painless separation of the connective tissue that holds the abdominals together. This separation may cause more pain in the lower back due to the increased load from lack of abdominal separation. Visit www.9monthsin9monthsout.com for exercises designed to help women keep their abdominals strong and flexible during pregnancy.

## *Do Your Kegels*

Kegel exercises should be a part of your daily routine, beginning in the second trimester. During the last months of pregnancy the growing fetus puts pressure on your bladder, which makes you feel the need to urinate frequently. Sometimes women limit their fluids when this happens, but it's absolutely essential that you keep your fluid intake high to stay hydrated. A better solution: Kegel exercises! These exercises strengthen the muscles around your urethra and can (and should) be done throughout your lifetime!

To perform a Kegel exercise, contract the muscles in your vagina, urethra, and anus — as if you were trying to hold back urine. Hold for five to seven seconds, then release. Repeat 10 to 20 times a day.

## *Common Exercise Complaints During the Second Trimester*

Many pregnant women feel rejuvenated after the first three months, they have more energy, are less tired, and can enjoy their workouts. However there can be a number of reasons you might want to modify your workout.

Exercise Modifications:
* Avoid exercises where Mom stays on her back for more than 60 seconds at a time (Vena Cava – Baby's Weight)
* Avoid balance exercises – relaxin hormone starts being released. Relaxin is a hormone produced during pregnancy that facilitates the birth process by causing a softening and lengthening of the cervix and the pubic symphysis.

# Relaxation and Stress Management for the Second Trimester

The second trimester should signal a rise in energy as your body and hormones begin to adjust to the baby. If you have been using the relaxation session in the first trimester, you'll be ready to begin to move on to the next step: Affirmations.

At this point, your baby is getting use to the sound of your voice and your partner's voice. We strongly advocate a "No-Negativity" rule with those around you.

No-Negativity includes:
* Listening to positive birth stories.
* Hearing loving voices, not those raised in anger.
* Reminding yourself to watch your phrasing and your tone when speaking aloud: the baby can hear you.

Creating this space provides you and your baby with more relaxation throughout the day. You are better able to listen to your body and interpret signs as good signs or those that should have you calling your healthcare provider. A woman in tune with her body will know when things are proceeding as expected in her pregnancy and will be better able to speak up for herself and participate in designing a Birth Plan.

## *Example Relaxation Technique*

Find a comfortable spot. Taking a few deep breaths in and up, out and down, just allowing you to unwind from the day. We're going to do just as we've done before.

*Imagine you are in the most relaxing space you know. It can be a warm summer's day on the beach, or a cool autumn afternoon near a mountain lake. Wherever your most relaxing space is. And as you lie motionless, imagine a warm white light just above your head. This white light is the most relaxing light you can imagine.*

*Allow the warmth of the light to flow down, over your forehead, feeling all little frown lines, all the little worry lines simply melt away. Letting the warmth flow down, over your eyes, your eyelids becoming warm and heavy, so heavy they don't even seem to want to open. They may flutter a little bit, but that's okay, just feel how heavy they are. Feeling the relaxation spread down over your face, letting all the muscles in your face unwind and relax. Allowing the warmth flow over your lips, and into your jaw. Feeling the warmth flow into your ears and around the back of your head. Feeling your whole head grow warm and relaxed.*

*The relaxation flows down the back of your neck now all the way through to your throat, feeling any blocks release and let go. Allowing the relaxation to spread down into your shoulders, feeling them drop a little. Feeling the warmth spread into your arms, down around your elbows, and into your forearms. Allowing the relaxation to wind around your wrists, flowing deep into your hands so that each and every finger relaxes more and more, more and more, as you go deeper and deeper into relaxation.*

*Now, allow the warmth to come back up to your throat and flow down into your chest. Feeling your heart relax. Feeling your lungs relax. Letting the relaxation flow all the way through to your back. Feeling your shoulder blades release and unwind. Feeling the warm white light flow all the way down your spine and around to your sides. Allowing the relaxation to flow deep into your stomach, feeling all the muscles, all the organs within your stomach release and let go. Allow the warm white light to flow around the baby, offering love and health, and then, let the warmth flow down into your hips, allowing your hips to release and unwind.*

*Allowing the warmth to flow down into the fronts of your thighs and all the way through to the backs. Down into the hollows of your knees, around to the knee itself. Feeling the warmth flow down into your shins, all the way through to your calves. Feeling the warmth flow down into your ankles and deep into the foot itself. Feeling each and every toe relax more and more, more and more, as you go deeper and deeper into relaxation.*

*Taking a deep breath in and up, out and down. Allowing your whole body to feel warm, safe and secure. Nice and relaxed. Just allowing yourself to go deeper and deeper and even deeper into relaxation.*

*Now, imagine yourself standing, and at the base of your feet is a beautiful stone stairway that leads downward into a very safe, valley of relaxation. This staircase will lead you to a profound state of deep, deep relaxation. We're going to go down these stairs now. Count backwards from ten to zero, each number will take you even deeper, and deeper, and even deeper into your relaxed state.*

*Ten. Taking that first step down now.*

*Nine, deeper and deeper.*

*Eight, way down now.*

*Seven, deeper… and deeper.*

*Six… deeper, feeling very relaxed now….*

*Five… deeper and deeper.*

*Four… you are going into a deep state of relaxation now.*

*Three, going deeper….*

*Two, relaxed even more, feeling very calm.*

*One. At the next number, you will enter this beautiful place of peace and tranquility called deep, deep relaxation. More relaxed and peaceful than you've ever known yourself to be.*

*And, zero.*

*Now, in a moment, count from five to one. And when you reach the count of one, your legs are going to be soooo relaxed, so heavy, that you will not be able to lift them.*

*Five – getting heavier and heavier now.*

*Four – more and more relaxed as you imagine the relaxation flowing through all the muscles in your legs.*

*Three – so deeply relaxed now as you imagine that relaxation flowing deep down into your bones.*

*Two – so relaxed, too relaxed to even move as you go from two… down to… one. Now, try to lift your legs and find with a bit of amusement that you cannot. They are just too heavy.*

*That's right, don't even try any more, they are just too relaxed.*

*Now, in a moment, count from five to one, one more time. Allow your eyes to become 100 times heavier than your legs just were. So heavy, they will not be able to open, no matter how much you try.*

*Five – feel the relaxation flowing around your eyes now.*

*Four – the relaxation crosses the bridge of your nose and flows thru the temples.*

*Three – feel the relaxation now flowing deep down into your eyes, all the way thru your head.*

*Two – so relaxed, too relaxed to open your eyes as you go from two down to one. So relaxed now, your eyes will not be able to open, but try. Try to open your eyes only when you are certain that you cannot.*

*That's right, don't even try anymore, they are just too heavy.*

*Very good. That's right. Just continuing to go deeper and deeper, relaxing.*

*Now, as you continue to listen to the sound of my voice, or even silently talk to yourself, we're going to repeat a few uplifting affirmations to help you and the baby thrive during this pregnancy. Remember that you are safe, secure, and relaxed here.*

*You are strong, confident and in control, already a loving mother.*

*You are giving your baby all that your baby needs.*

*You're eating healthy and consuming just the right amount of calories for you both to share.*

*You're drinking your large glasses of water all day long, avoiding any temptations.*

*You are sleeping soundly and deeply at night, feeling restful when you wake.*

*You have all the energy you need to get everything done in a day.*

*Your body is strong and energetic.*

*Your baby is growing and thriving each and every day.*

*Your cravings lean to healthier foods, fruits, vegetables, all the things that help make your baby strong and healthy. You shy away from high sugar or high salt foods, finding your body craves fresher foods, more organic.*

*You look forward to getting a daily walk in, or your workouts, feeling stronger and healthier.*

*You are taking your vitamins, feeling stronger for taking them and knowing good nutrients are flowing through you to your baby.*

*Your body is growing and adjusting exactly as it needs to, allowing room for the baby.*

*People are naturally telling you only good stories.*

*You carry an inner smile with you wherever you go.*

*Your body is naturally maintaining the correct weight for you and your baby. You are gaining the appropriate amount of weight to help nourish you baby.*

Taking a deep breath in and up, out and down. Just continuing to go deeper and deeper, relaxing. As you continue to listen to the sound of the music, simply allow your body to relax to sleep. A deep, warm, comfortable, healing sleep. Letting the rest and relaxation flow from you to baby. Simply… drifting… relaxing… sleeping deeply now.

## Massage in the Second Trimester

Now is a good time to start working on the abdominal muscles in more ways than one. Massage on the muscles that are starting to pull tight across your growing belly can help ease feelings of tightness and help relax the lower back. It also helps cut down on diastasis or the separation of the abs as your belly gets bigger, and increase blood flow to the area which can in turn help to keep the skin soft and supple to help cut down on stretch marks.

## *Positioning*

After the 13th week of pregnancy it is recommended to avoid lying flat on your back to avoid Supine Hypotensive Syndrome, which is when the uterus and its contents compress the blood vessel that returns blood from the lower half of the body.

It may not be possible at this point to lie on your stomach comfortably any more. Some tables have a cut out to hang your belly through but there is some controversy about whether it is a good idea to use these tables as there is nothing supporting the weight of the uterus and may put too much strain on the back. You may find that using pillows above and below your belly while lying face down works for you for a while until your stomach grows too large for that as well.

As always, pay attention to the signals your body is giving you. If it feels wrong, it probably is.

## Conclusion

Your second trimester is winding down. You've most likely been energetic and feeling the best you have felt in a long time. Now enjoy the final weeks of your pregnancy, the prepping and nesting phase.

# Third Trimester

You're now in the home stretch! You've been eating healthy choices and getting in exercise. You've been mentally and emotionally preparing yourself with positive thoughts and affirmations. You've been poked and prodded and are *really* ready for this baby to be born. If this is your first child, enjoy these last few months – spend time with your partner, your pets, your friends, and your family. Things will change, and it'll be worth every minute.

## Third Trimester Development

| Timing | Developments |
|---|---|
| *Notes* | Due to increased blood volume, symptoms of carpal tunnel syndrome can appear.<br><br>As the weight of the uterus increases, the uterosacral ligament pulls on the sacrum increasing the natural curve in the lower back and can cause soreness and muscle spasms.<br><br>Round ligament pain can be triggered by sudden movements and can be painful enough in the lower abdomen to be pretty scary. Pulling knees in towards the chest can help relieve pain. |
| *Twenty-Nine to Thirty-Five Weeks* | Your baby's eyes can now open and close and can sense light changes.<br><br>The lanugo is starting to disappear from the baby's face. Your baby's hearing is getting better and the baby can now hear the outside world quite well over the sound of your heartbeat. Talk to your baby! Play your favorite CD!<br><br>The baby exercises by kicking and stretching and can now make grasping motions.<br><br>Your baby likes to suck its thumb!<br><br>The bones are getting stronger, limbs fatter, and the skin has a healthy glow.<br><br>The brain is now forming its different regions. The brain and nerves are directing bodily functions.<br><br>Taste buds are developing. |

| | |
|---|---|
| | Your baby may now hiccup, cry, taste sweet and sour, and respond to pain, light, and sound. |
| | If you are having a boy, his testicles have fully descended from his abdomen into his scrotum. |
| | By the end of the 35th week, your baby will be approximately 16 to 18 inches long and weigh about 4 pounds. |
| *Thirty-Six to Forty Weeks* | Your baby is now gaining about a half pound each week, and is getting fatter (adipose tissue layer developing) and its skin is less rumpled. |
| | The baby is getting ready for birth and is settling into the fetal position with its head down against the cervix, its legs tucked up to its chest, and its knees against its nose. |
| | Your antibodies to disease are beginning to flow rapidly through the placenta. The rapid flow of blood through the umbilical cord keeps it taunt, which prevents tangles. |
| | Your baby is beginning to develop sleeping patterns. |
| | The baby will continue to kick and punch although it will move lower in your abdomen to under your pelvis (this is called "lightening" or "the baby has dropped"). You will also feel your baby roll around as it gets too cramped inside the uterus for much movement. |
| | Your baby's lungs are now mature and your baby will have a great chance of survival if born a little early. |
| | The bones of the baby's head are soft and flexible to ease the process through the birth canal. |
| | Your baby is now about 20 inches long and weighs approximately 6 to 9 pounds. |
| | Your baby may be born between the 37th and 41st week of pregnancy. Only 5% of babies are born on their due date and most first pregnancies go past their due date. |

Table 5. Third Trimester Development.

# Your Birth Plan

A birth plan is a simple, clear, one-page statement of your preferences for the birth of your baby. Having a copy for every person involved in the birth will help each person understand each other and work out communication issues before the big day. Because there are so many aspects of birth to consider, it is best not to wait until the last minute to create your plan. You will want to discuss it with those who will support and care for you.

Try to remember: *Be flexible. Deviations may be necessary for your health and the health of your baby.* You will also want to remember the goal: the safe birth of your little bundle of joy. Keeping this goal in mind, the following step-by-step guide will help you create your birth plan.

Keep in mind that every birth is different and that a "normal" birth may have a wide range of definitions; use wording like "birth preferences," "our wishes for childbirth," "as long as birth progresses normally," or "unless there is an emergency."

A written plan is handy as it will help you and your partner be better prepared during all the activity that happens during birth. You can print off a sample birth plan available on our website at www.9monthsin9monthsout.com.

*In general, here are the areas you might want to include in your plan:*
- Names of the people you would like in attendance during your labor and birth: your partner, midwife, doula, etc. A doula is a woman who provides non-medical support during labor and birth.
- Music, lighting, film/photography, and clothing preferences.
- Types of birthing equipment you'd like to bring or try, e.g., birthing balls, stools, etc.
- Type of birthing positions you'd like to try (semi-reclining, side, kneeling, squatting or whatever feels the most comfortable).
- Pain relief method of your preference: acupressure, self-hypnosis, medication, massage, etc.
- What you would like to occur during a vaginal birth or c-section (do you want to see/touch/have your partner see/touch, etc.)

Other items to include in your plan are rooming in, breast/formula fed, and more. We've tried to make it easy by providing you a quick form on our website (www.9monthsin9monthsout.com) to fill out and check off before sharing it with your healthcare provider and partner.

During childbirth, many women feel like they are losing control. Your birth plan helps you to be confident and trust in your body and helps you feel part of the decision making even if unexpected events occur. Plan for the unexpected. Use positive language instead of negative verbiage like "I don't want, or I want to avoid…'.

Bring your birth plan to one of your visits in the third trimester and discuss/review with your healthcare provider.

Make sure you have a copy of your birth plan in your hospital bag! You don't want to stress out because you forgot your copy.

# Medical Considerations

You'll have more healthcare provider visits to check you and your baby and to make sure everything is progressing normally. Look at these appointments as a great way to hear your baby's heartbeat, see your progress in your pregnancy and to have all of your questions addressed.

And, time for one last test! Group B Strep (GBS) or group B strep is one of many common bacteria that live in the human body without causing harm in healthy people. GBS develops in the intestine, so sometimes it is present and sometimes it is not. GBS can be found in your intestine, rectum, and vagina in about 2 of every 10 pregnant women near the time of birth. GBS is NOT a sexually transmitted disease, and it does not cause discharge, itching, or other symptoms.

At the time of birth, babies are exposed to the GBS bacteria if it is present in the vagina, which can result in pneumonia or a blood infection. Full-term babies who are born to mothers who carry GBS in the vagina at the time of birth have a 1 in 200 chance of getting sick from GBS during the first few days after being born. Occasionally, moms can get a postpartum infection in the uterus as well.

Around your 35th to 36th week, during a regular prenatal visit, your healthcare provider will collect a sample by touching the outer part of your vagina and just inside the anus with a sterile Q-tip. If GBS grows in the culture that is sent to the lab from that Q-tip sample, your healthcare provider will discuss the results at your next prenatal visit to talk about your plan of care in labor.

If your GBS culture is positive within four to five weeks before you give birth, your healthcare provider will recommend that you receive antibiotics during labor. GBS is very sensitive to antibiotics and is easily removed from the vagina. A few intravenous doses given up to four hours before birth almost always prevents your baby from picking up the bacteria during the birth.

Although GBS is easy to remove from the vagina, it is not easy to remove from the intestine where it lives normally and without harm to you. Although GBS is not dangerous to you or your baby before birth, if you take antibiotics before you are in labor, GBS will return to the vagina from the intestine, as soon as you stop taking the medication. Therefore, it is best to take penicillin during labor when it can best help you and your baby. The one exception is that, occasionally, GBS can cause a urinary tract infection during pregnancy. If you get a urinary tract infection, it should be treated at the time it is diagnosed, and then you should receive antibiotics again when you are in labor.

Babies who get sick from infection with GBS almost always show signs and symptoms in the first 24 hours after birth. Symptoms include difficulty with breathing (including grunting or having poor color), problems maintaining temperature (too cold or too hot), or extreme sleepiness that interferes with nursing.

If the infection is caught early and your baby is full-term, most babies will completely recover with intravenous antibiotic treatment. Of the babies who get sick, about one in six can have serious complications. Some very seriously ill babies will die. In the large majority of cases, if you carry GBS in the vagina at the time of birth and if you are given intravenous antibiotics in labor, the risk of your baby getting sick is 1 in 4,000.

Penicillin or a penicillin-type medication is the antibiotic recommended for preventing GBS infection. Women who carry GBS at the time of birth and who are allergic to penicillin can receive different antibiotics during labor. Be sure to tell your healthcare provider if you are allergic to penicillin and what symptoms you had when you got that allergic reaction. If your penicillin allergy is mild, you will be offered one type of antibiotic, and if it is severe, you will be offered a different one.

It is important to remember that GBS is typically not harmful to you or your baby before you are in labor. You want your healthcare provider to conduct this test to keep you and your baby safe.

Think of these appointments as a great time to get more familiar with your baby and the process of birth in addition to your child birth classes. Make sure you're asking questions as they come up. While your appointments may be short and sweet, they can also be informative and help you plan.

# Nutrition in the Third Trimester

Your third trimester marks a time of rapid fetal growth, and if Mom isn't careful, rapid weight gain for her in the buttocks, thighs and belly. Moms traditionally gain 10-18 pounds in this last trimester. Nutrients are extremely important and it is necessary to avoid empty calories – the ones that taste super good yet provide no nutritional value.

*Follow these simple nutrition tips:*

**Switch to Mini-Meals** – As you and your baby are getting bigger you may not feel like eating three regular meals. However, it is still necessary for you to eat a well-balanced diet with sufficient calories. So, switch to five or six lighter meals or snacks spread throughout the day.

**Drink Plenty of Water** – Some women feel they could describe what every restroom in the city looks like by now and it's no wonder. Staying properly hydrated is very important for you and your baby. In fact, it helps prevent constipation, keeps swelling down and may help reduce stretch marks. So keep on downing those 8 to 10 cups of water a day!

**Make Sure You Continue to Get Your Iron** – Faster rate of growth for Mom and Baby equals the need for more blood, and therefore, more iron! Meat sources of iron contain the heme form of iron, which is well absorbed in the body. Vegetarians are at greater risk of iron deficiency in pregnancy than meat eaters.

**Vitamin C** – Vitamin C increases the absorption of the non-heme iron found in vegetable sources. Vitamin C foods include fresh fruits such as oranges, grapefruits, kiwis and strawberries. This nutrient is also important for tissue repair and can aid in recovery after giving birth.

**Vitamin D** – Since the baby's bones are developing and hardening, you need extra calcium. You can actually get vitamin D from the sun and 15 minutes a day is enough. Other sources include milk, fish, and fortified cereal. Strive for 1,000 IU of vitamin D per day.

**Folic Acid** – Your body and your baby need folic acid to produce and repair DNA and allow it to function. It is also important for the production of red blood cells. You should get 800 mcg a day. Folic acid is essential for a healthy baby and helps in the development of the fetal brain and spine. Women should take 800 mcg of folic acid every day throughout their pregnancy and need to take a prenatal vitamin to meet this requirement. Some excellent sources of folic acid include dried beans, tofu, peanuts and peanut butter, as well as fortified cereals. Many types of bread are now also fortified with folic acid. Folic acid can also be found in many dark green vegetables, corn, cantaloupe, squash and beets.

**Calcium** – Your baby's growing bones need more calcium, and his/her growing muscles and tissues need protein. Calcium is one of the most important minerals you will need during pregnancy. The current recommended amount of calcium intake during pregnancy is 1,200 mg a day. That's an increase of 400 mg a day over your usual needs. An increase in dairy products such as skim milk, cheese, yogurt, pudding and ice milk, is an easy way to consume lots of calcium. There are also many good non-dairy sources of calcium, including salmon, kale, broccoli, beans and calcium-fortified orange juice.

**Omega-3s** – For rapid brain development, your baby needs omega-3 fatty acids and zinc. Omega-3's are essential fatty acids (EFAs) and affect development of the fetus. One of the most important EFAs is called docosahexaenoic acid (DHA), which is found in fish. DHA has a biological role in the structure and function of the brain, retina and nervous system. The brain of the developing baby grows rapidly during the last trimester and is dependent upon the mother's intake of DHA. Clinical studies have shown that increasing the mother's intake of DHA through supplementation with fish oil (oil from fish such as tuna is high in DHA) results in higher blood levels of DHA in the newborn. The brain continues to grow and develop rapidly for the first year and an adequate supply of DHA is necessary over this period.

Eating a nutrient-rich diet can also help your body recover and repair itself after you give birth. Fatty acids are stored in the body and can be released and delivered to the fetus when needed. However, pregnancy causes a decline in the EFA and LCP status of the mother. DHA concentration drops dramatically during pregnancy and may develop into a deficiency, leading to premature births and low birth weight babies. The mother's ability to supply DHA may be insufficient to meet the needs of the fetus if she has inadequate stores and/or intake.

**Vitamin B12 & B6** – Vitamin B12, found in animal products, is essential for proper nerve and brain functioning for both you and your baby. This is of special concern for women who are vegetarians. Vitamin B12 can be found in fortified soymilk and/or soy meat replacements, as well as vitamin supplements. You'll also need more vitamin B6 in your diet to help you metabolize that extra protein.

**Protein** – During pregnancy, the body conserves protein, especially in the last half of pregnancy when the demand is greatest. Protein is stored in the maternal tissues, with the greatest storage occurring in the last 10 weeks of pregnancy. The total amount of protein needed for the fetus, placenta, amniotic fluid, uterus, blood, and extracellular fluid has been estimated at 925 grams for a normal 270-day pregnancy, with 760 grams accumulated in the last 20 weeks of pregnancy.

Maternal protein deficiency can have serious fetal consequences. Metabolism is altered if the quantity and/or quality of protein is inadequate. Even though amino acids are transported from mother to fetus across a concentration gradient, if the supply is inadequate in the mother, the fetus will be deficient.

Protein can easily be found in animal products including meats, milk and eggs. Some plant foods, such as legumes, seeds and cereal grains, can also provide high quality protein. It is more beneficial if you combine one food from two of these categories in the form of such dishes as hummus, split pea soup, bean tacos or even a peanut butter sandwich.

**Fiber and Carbohydrates** – Total fiber consists of dietary fiber and functional fiber, two very different types of fiber. Dietary fiber consists of non-digestible carbohydrates and lignins that are part of plants, such as cellulose, pectin, gums, hemicellulose, beta-glucans, oligosaccharides, fructans, and lignans. Dietary fiber can be found in bran, grains, vegetables, legumes, seeds, and nuts. Functional fibers are isolated non-digestible carbohydrates that have beneficial physiological effects in humans such as pectin, gums, chitin, polydextrose, inulin, and indigestible dextrins. Sources of functional fiber include grains, vegetables, and other plant foods.

The RDA for carbohydrates during pregnancy is 175 grams per day, which accounts for both maternal and fetal glucose needs. The median intake of carbohydrates is approximately 180 grams per day to 230 grams per day, which is within the recommendations. Following a low-carbohydrate diet is not appropriate during pregnancy.

Remember, the healthier your choices are now, the less weight you will have to lose post pregnancy. And, the healthier you eat, with variety, the better your baby will develop.

# Exercise in the Third Trimester

As your pregnancy progresses, the extra weight and its distribution can place stress on your joints and muscles, especially in the lower back and pelvis. Women might also have problems with circulation, causing leg cramps and dizziness. Adapt your exercise regimen accordingly in the third trimester, depending on how you feel and switch to low-impact activities, such as walking, swimming, and indoor cycling. In fact, some women are so fatigued and have so much difficulty moving around that they aren't able to exercise at all during the third trimester, but if you can, keep it up. Studies show that women who exercise during the third trimester achieve the greatest benefits from that exercise: reduced fat gain, shorter and less complicated labor and birth process, and shorter recovery after giving birth from exercise.

If you are still engaging in rigorous workouts, such as cycling or step exercises, this would be a good time to shift to less strenuous activities — and those that don't require careful balance. As your baby has grown, your center of gravity has further shifted. You also may have less oxygen available, so reduce the pace of your routines, or stop altogether if you become breathless.

As you go through your third trimester, keep the following potential modifications and tips in mind:

- Keep doing your pelvic floor exercises (Kegels), even if you're not able to do anything else. But be careful as you get up from the floor and move slowly to avoid injury.
- As with the second trimester, avoid overstretching. And if you haven't already discontinued outdoor cycling, now is definitely the time to begin cycling indoors.
- In addition to needing a new sports bra, you may need a support belt or belly brace.

> **When Not To Exercise in the Third Trimester**
>
> Discontinue any exercise if any of the following apply:
>
> - If you have pregnancy-induced high blood pressure.
> - If you have asthma.
> - If you experience bleeding during the second trimester.
> - If you have a history of late miscarriage.

## Common Exercise Complaints During the Third Trimester

- Tiredness or lack of sleep due to increased pressure of the uterus on the bladder or due to pressure on other internal organs
- Sciatica from excess weight putting pressure on the back
- Breasts are sore preparing for breast-feeding

*Exercise Modifications:*
- All supine (lying down, face up) exercises are out now
- Watch exercises that require balance
- Ideal cardio methods are water aerobics, elliptical, bike and walking
- Ideal resistance training are machines or bands

# Relaxation in the Third Trimester

As you move into the final few months of your pregnancy, you'll start to feel as if you're carrying more weight than you actually are. Hopefully, with the help of all the information in this book, you've found your pregnancy to be smooth and flowing. For the final few months, we're going to add another layer into your relaxation sessions. We're starting to prepare you for the actual process of birth.

Now, you may have chosen to take any one of the childbirth classes offered. You may be focusing on a natural birth, epidural for pain management or even a c-section. The goal of this relaxation session is to help to keep you and your baby calm regardless of what method of birth you've chosen to experience. We recommend you start using this relaxation around week 34.

Find a comfortable spot. Taking a few deep breaths in and up, out and down. Just allow yourself to unwind from the day. We're going to do just as we've done before.

*Imagine you are in the most relaxing space you know. It can be a warm summer's day on the beach, or a cool autumn afternoon near a mountain lake. Wherever your most relaxing space is. And as you lie motionless, imagine a warm white light just above your head. This white light is the most relaxing light you can imagine.*

*Allow the warmth of the light to flow down, over your forehead, feeling all little frown lines, all the little worry lines simply melt away. Letting the warmth flow down, over your eyes, your eyelids becoming warm and heavy, so heavy they don't even seem to want to open. They may flutter a little bit, but that's okay, just feel how heavy they are. Feeling the relaxation spread down over your face, letting all the muscles in your face unwind and relax. Allowing the warmth flow over your lips, and into your jaw. Feeling the warmth flow into your ears and around the back of your head. Feeling your whole head grow warm and relaxed.*

*The relaxation flows down the back of your neck now all the way through to your throat, feeling any blocks release and let go. Allowing the relaxation to spread down into your shoulders, feeling them drop a little. Feeling the warmth spread into your arms, down around your elbows, and into your forearms. Allowing the relaxation to wind around your wrists, flowing deep into your hands so that each and every finger relaxes more and more, more and more, as you go deeper and deeper into relaxation.*

*Now, allow the warmth to come back up to your throat and flow down into your chest. Feeling your heart relax. Feeling your lungs relax. Letting the relaxation flow all the way through to your back.*

*Feeling your shoulder blades release and unwind. Feeling the warm white light flow all the way down your spine and around to your sides. Allowing the relaxation to flow deep into your stomach, feeling all the muscles, all the organs within your stomach release and let go. Allow the warm white light to flow around the baby, offering love and health, and then, let the warmth flow down into your hips, allowing your hips to release and unwind.*

*Allowing the warmth to flow down into the fronts of your thighs and all the way through to the backs. Down into the hollows of your knees, around to the knee itself. Feeling the warmth flow down into your shins, all the way through to your calves. Feeling the warmth flow down into your ankles and deep into the foot itself. Feeling each and every toe relax more and more, more and more, as you go deeper and deeper into relaxation.*

*Taking a deep breath in and up, out and down. Allowing your whole body to feel warm, safe and secure. Nice and relaxed. Just allowing yourself to go deeper and deeper and even deeper into relaxation.*

*Now, imagine yourself standing, and at the base of your feet is a beautiful stone stairway that leads downward into a very safe valley of relaxation. This staircase will lead you to a profound state of deep, deep relaxation. Go down these stairs now, and count backwards from ten to zero. Each number will take you even deeper, and deeper, and even deeper into your relaxed state.*

*Ten. Taking that first step down now.*

*Nine, deeper and deeper.*

*Eight, way down now.*

*Seven, deeper ... and deeper.*

*Six... deeper, feeling very relaxed now....*

*Five… deeper and deeper.*

*Four… you are going into a deep state of relaxation now.*

*Three, going deeper….*

*Two, relaxed even more, feeling very calm.*

*One. At the next number, you will enter this beautiful place of peace and tranquility called deep, deep relaxation. More relaxed and peaceful than you've ever known yourself to be.*

*And, zero.*

*Now, in a moment, count from five to one. And when you reach the count of one, your legs are going to be soooo relaxed, so heavy, that you will not be able to lift them.*

*Five – getting heavier and heavier now.*

*Four – more and more relaxed as you imagine the relaxation flowing through all the muscles in your legs.*

*Three – so deeply relaxed now as you imagine that relaxation flowing deep down into your bones.*

*Two – so relaxed, too relaxed to even move as you go from two… down to… one. Now, try to lift your legs and find with a bit of amusement that you cannot. They are just too heavy.*

*That's right, don't even try any more, they are just too relaxed.*

*Now, in a moment, count from five to one, one more time. Allow your eyes to become 100 times heavier than your legs just were. So heavy, they will not be able to open, no matter how much you try.*

*Five – feel the relaxation flowing around your eyes now.*

*Four – the relaxation crosses the bridge of your nose and flows thru the temples.*

*Three – feel the relaxation now flowing deep down into your eyes, all the way thru your head.*

*Two – so relaxed, too relaxed to open your eyes as you go from two down to one. So relaxed now, your eyes will not be able to open, but try. Try to open your eyes only when you are certain that you cannot.*

*That's right, don't even try anymore, they are just too heavy.*

*Very good. That's right. Just continuing to go deeper and deeper, relaxing.*

*Now, as you continue to listen to the sound of my voice, or even silently talk to yourself, we're going to repeat our affirmations to help you and the baby thrive during these final few months of pregnancy. And now, we're adding in all those suggestions you need to have a safe and relaxed delivery of a healthy, happy baby. Remember you are safe, secure, and relaxed here.*

*You are strong, confident and in control, already a loving mother.*

*You are giving your baby all that your baby needs.*

*You're eating healthy and consuming just the right amount of calories for you both to share.*

*You're drinking your large glasses of water all day long, avoiding any temptations.*

*You are sleeping soundly and deeply at night, feeling restful when you wake.*

*You have all the energy you need to get everything done in a day.*

*Your body is strong and energetic.*

*Your baby is growing and thriving each and every day.*

*Your cravings lean to healthier foods, fruits, vegetables, all the things that help make your baby strong and healthy. You shy away from high sugar or high salt foods, finding your body craves fresher foods, more organic.*

*You look forward to getting a daily walk in, or your workouts, feeling stronger and healthier.*

*You are taking your vitamins, feeling stronger for taking them and knowing good nutrients are flowing thru you to your baby.*

*Your body is growing and adjusting exactly as it needs to, allowing room for the baby.*

*People are naturally telling you only good stories.*

*You carry an inner smile with you wherever you go.*

*Your body is naturally maintaining the correct weight for you and your baby. You are gaining the appropriate amount of weight to help nourish you baby.*

*Your body is readjusting at the correct time. The baby is turning into the optimal position for birth just as needed. Your muscles flow like ribbons, expanding and contracting as needed to allow your body to prepare and deliver this baby.*

*Contractions, when they come, ripple through your body with ease, feeling just as if you were using your muscles to lift a weight in the gym, or flow through a yoga pose. There is only movement, acknowledgement of movement and a knowing that the body is preparing for delivery.*

*You are at peace with the process of birth; it is a natural cycle. Your body simply responds in flowing motions, allowing the baby to be born with ease.*

Taking a deep breath in and up, out and down. Just continuing to go deeper and deeper, relaxing. As you continue to listen to the sound of the music, simply allow your body to relax to sleep. A deep, warm, comfortable, healing sleep. Letting the rest and relaxation flow from you to your baby. Simply… drifting… relaxing… sleeping deeply now.

## Massage in the Third Trimester

*In the third trimester some of the less comfortable side effects of pregnancy that can be relieved by massage are one or more of the following:*

- Swelling of the feet, ankles and hands can appear or increase. Elevating the feet and massage can both help to alleviate this. Add a fresh lemon or lemon juice to your water to help alleviate swelling.
- Due to increased blood volume, symptoms of carpal tunnel syndrome can appear. Massage can help to move the circulation through the area and decrease the nerve symptoms in hands and wrists.
- As the weight of the uterus increases, the uterosacral ligament pulls on the sacrum increasing the natural curve in the lower back and can cause soreness and muscle spasms. There are back supports on the market that decrease the pressure on the back. Massage can help to ease the accumulation of tension in the area, which may cut down on the severity and frequency of spasms.

Remember that round ligament pain in your lower abdomen can be triggered by sudden movements and can be painful and scary. Check with your healthcare provider to make sure nothing more serious is going on. If your physician or midwife confirms your discomfort is indeed round ligament pain, there are a few things that can ease the pain. Pulling knees in towards the chest can help relieve pain. A warm bath can be helpful but avoid excessive heat. A moderate temperature on a heating pad is fine for a short period of time. Lying on your side with a pillow under the stomach and one between the legs can ease discomfort. Avoiding sudden movements, and pushing yourself up from the side instead of sitting straight up can cut down on the sharp pains.

## *Positioning*

While in the second trimester positioning was something you evaluated by what felt right, in the third trimester it is now important to use alternative positions.

Here are some of the alternative positions your therapist may use to avoid putting undue pressure on your baby.

**Left Lateral Tilt** – Using pillows or props under the right side of the body, tilt the weight towards your left to take the pressure off of the major blood flow

**Fowler's Position** – Elevate the upper body for a "semi-reclining" position with a prop under the knees for comfort

**Side Lying** – The side lying position is made more comfortable with a pillow under the head, another to prop up the top leg and one may be used to support the belly as well

## *Infant Massage*

Now is the time to start learning infant massage. A massage therapist trained in infant massage is typically not going to work on your baby, but will teach you some routines to use with your baby yourself.

The physical act of touching between the baby and parents can help with the bonding process. Studies have shown that babies who receive touch therapy gain weight faster and exhibit less failure to thrive. The results with premature babies were exemplary. Some say that infant massage can enhance a baby's ability to learn by stimulating them through tactile touch.

There are different methods of infant massage. There is the Swedish method and the Indian method. The Indian method consists of squeezes, twisting motions and stroking the extremities away from the heart. The intention has to do with removing negative energy from the body. While the intentions are good, the Swedish method argues that this method is potentially damaging to the valves in those delicate baby veins. Damaged valves can result in varicose veins. In a Swedish massage, the strokes are all in the direction moving toward the heart. If the concept of removing negative energy is something that is important to you, it is highly recommended that any stroke directed away from the heart be a light one. Those who believe in the ability to move energy around agree that it is the intent, not the amount of pressure that is important in removing negative energy.

## Conclusion

It's almost time! You've finished up all the tests your healthcare provider recommended. You've eaten as healthy as you could and kept up with an exercise routine. You've listened to your baby's heartbeat and saw your baby via ultrasound. We all love having the ultrasound pictures to share. Now, it's time to meet your baby. But first, a little work with the birthing process....

# 9 Months Out

# Your Birth Day:
# What to Expect During Labor

It is normal for you to feel both excited and scared about labor and birth. Be sure to have all of your questions answered about labor and birth during your weekly visits beginning at 36 weeks. If you attended childbirth classes, be sure to ask your healthcare provider questions you may have that were not clearly explained in class.

## *Preparing Your Other Children*

If you already have children at home, preparing your child or children ahead of time for the birth of their new sister or brother will help them adjust when the baby is born.

Assess the needs of the older child and do your best to meet those needs. Help them feel safe and secure. All the changes in your family can cause some children to feel anxious.

*Below are some practical suggestions:*

- Tell your child about his or her "babyhood". Share a story of their childhood together – how he or she started out "just" like their new brother or sister.
- Show your child photos of special events or moments of him or her as a baby.
- Take your child with you to your prenatal visits. Have your child listen to the baby's heartbeat and feel the baby kick within your tummy.
- Give your child a new doll or stuffed animal so he or she can practice caring for a "baby" too.
- Make arrangements for your child's care while you are in the hospital. Discuss these arrangements with your child well before the baby's due date. Make it a fun sleep over!

- Prepare the baby's bedroom or sleeping area well in advance, so your child can adjust. Let them help!
- Place a baby photo of the older child at the child's eye level in the baby's room or where the family spends the most time.
- Talk with your child about what the new brother or sister will be like. Use books that show pictures of babies and discuss what babies can and cannot do.
- Develop a method of long-distance contact with the older child before going to the hospital. Some ideas are: call the child by phone so he/she will get used to the sound of your voice on the phone; write notes to the child to ask him or her to do small jobs; make a video or audio recording of you reading a story to the child.

*Involve your child in preparations for the new baby. If the child wants to, let him or her:*
- Help you pack your suitcase for the hospital.
- Help select the new baby's name.
- Help pick out the new baby's coming home clothes.
- Make the baby's homecoming a special event for the whole family.
- Have a birthday cake and family birthday party to celebrate the new baby when you return home from the hospital.
- If the child wants to, let him or her help making birth announcements by drawing pictures, etc.
- Ask your older child to pass out something special to friends announcing the baby's birth.
- Arrange for your children to exchange gifts. Ask your older child to pick out a special gift for the baby.
- Once the new baby comes home:
- Involve your child in caring for the new baby. Have him or her bring the diapers to you as you change the baby. Engage them in helping dress and burp the baby. If the older sibling is not interested in helping with activities, provide an activity for him or her to enjoy while you care for the new addition.
- Show the older child how to interact with the baby. Have them smile and talk with the baby and explain how the baby enjoys this. Have the older sibling hold the baby with supervision.

- Share some (but not all) toys with the baby – let the older child keep the toys that are very special to him or her. Have a drawer or a place in the baby's room for some of his or her toys.

*Things you can do for the older child:*
- Bathe the new baby and older child at the same time if older child doesn't object.
- Have a learning session for your older child. Undress your baby, talk about the different parts and functions of the body – using correct terminology. Curiosity often can be satisfied by direct observation. Let your older child touch the baby as you emphasize "gently." Use the words "don't touch" as little as possible.
- Allow older child to verbalize negative feelings toward the baby or you.
- While you are in the hospital, make sure the older child stays with someone who they feel very comfortable with. It will make this time less traumatic.

*Once you come home with the new baby make sure you continue to:*
- Talk, hold and show affection to the sibling whenever you notice or sense signs of jealously or regressive behavior. Some children regress after a younger sibling is born. The areas that may be affected include eating, toileting, crying and sleeping. Don't punish the older sibling because of his/her regression; rather, reassure the child and offer praise for his or her "big brother" or "big sister" actions and behavior.
- Praise positive behavior; ignore negative behavior. Reward only those behaviors you want to continue.
- Parents may want to use a task chart with gold stars to encourage positive behavior.
- Remind the older child that he or she is special too.
- There is certain space in the home that belongs to the sibling exclusively. Parents and baby should respect this space.
- Reinforce your child's role in the family, especially as the older sibling.
- Give your older child "seniority" by providing special jobs at home so he or she can contribute to the family.
- Spend as much time as possible alone with your older child throughout the day and especially at bedtime.

- Purchase small gifts for the older child. When visitors bring a gift for the new baby, give previously purchased gift(s) to the older child to make him/her feel celebrated as well.
- When friends come to visit the new baby, parents should include the older child in conversations or activities. For example, the older child could show the new baby to visitors.
- Provide a planned activity for your older child while caring for the baby.
- Plan activities outside of home with the older child only. There should be a routine weekly outing for the sibling (park, restaurant, library, etc.).
- Encourage independent behavior (at play, dressing or toileting), as appropriate for the child's age. Some children enjoy knowing they are more capable of caring for themselves and seek ways of becoming more independent.
- Parents may want to use a task chart for children when they help with jobs around the house and with tasks associated with the new baby.

## True Labor versus False Labor

*Is this it? Am I in labor? Is the baby finally coming?* These are the questions that moms-to-be ponder on a daily basis when they are close to their due date. In the last several weeks of pregnancy, you may notice that your abdomen gets hard and then soft again. As you get closer to your delivery date, you may find that this becomes more uncomfortable or even painful at times. These irregular cramps are called Braxton-Hicks contractions. You may also experience contractions following a vaginal exam or intercourse and they may occur more frequently when you are physically active. Again, these are Braxton-Hicks contractions and will eventually subside.

*If you begin to experience contractions:*
- Remember to use your Reverse Pattern Breathing Technique found on page 96 to help stay calm.
- Drink one liter of water in an hour's time.
- Take two extra-strength Tylenol (acetaminophen).
- Soak in a warm, not hot, bath.

*Special Note: If the contractions are false labor pains, they will begin to go away. If the contractions are true labor, they will get closer in frequency and more intense.*

False labor can occur just at the time when labor is expected to start, and it is sometimes difficult to tell true from false labor. Don't be upset or embarrassed if you react by thinking that labor has begun. Sometimes the difference can only be determined by a vaginal exam. Always feel comfortable calling your healthcare provider to discuss your symptoms. Timing of contractions in false labor often are irregular and do not consistently develop a close pattern (Braxton-Hicks contractions), but sometimes you can be fooled!

## What are the Stages of Labor?

The average labor lasts 12 to 24 hours for a first birth and is usually shorter for other subsequent births. Labor happens in three stages.

**First Stage** - The first stage is the longest part of labor and can last many hours. It begins when your cervix starts to open and ends when it is completely open (fully dilated) at 10 centimeters. When the cervix dilates from zero to five centimeters, contractions get stronger as time progresses. Mild contractions begin at 15 to 20 minutes apart and last 45 to 60 seconds. The contractions become more regular until they are less than five minutes apart. When the cervix dilates from five to eight centimeters (called the Active Phase), contractions get stronger and are about three minutes apart, lasting about 60 to 90 seconds.

---

### Tips to Help with the Active Phase

- Try changing your position. You may want to try getting on your hands and knees – this helps ease the discomfort of back labor. You also may want to use the birthing ball which also helps ease back discomfort and helps baby "move down" into the pelvis and provides you partner easy access to your lower back for back massage and counter pressure.
- Soak in a warm tub or take a warm shower.
- Continue practicing breathing and relaxation techniques.
- Stay out of bed!

---

You may have a backache and increased bleeding from your vagina (show). Your mood may become more serious as you focus on the hard work of dealing with the contractions. You will also depend more on your support person and your healthcare provider/nurse-midwife.

If your bag of waters ruptures, the next contractions may be much stronger. When the cervix dilates from 8 to 10 centimeters (called the Transition Phase), contractions are two to three minutes apart and last about one minute. You may feel pressure on your rectum and your backache may feel worse. Bleeding from your vagina will be heavier.

It may help to practice breathing and relaxation techniques such as massage or listening to soothing music. Focus on taking one contraction at a time. Remember that each contraction brings you closer to holding your baby!

**Second Stage** - The second stage of labor begins when your cervix is fully dilated at 10 centimeters. This stage continues until your baby passes through the birth canal or vagina and is born. This stage may last two hours or longer if this is your first baby.

Contractions may feel different – they will slow to two to five minutes apart and last from about 60 to 90 seconds. You will feel a strong urge to push with your contractions. Try to rest as much as possible between intervals of pushing.

If you do not have an urge to push when you are completely dilated, this is Mother Nature's way of giving you a resting period and to conserve your energy for when it is time to push. Take advantage of this time and close your eyes, visualizing your baby in your arms!

*Here are some helpful hints for pushing:*
- Try several positions: squatting, getting on your hands and knees, lying on your side.
- Take deep breaths in and out before and after each contraction.
- Curl your body into a "C" position or into the push as much as possible. Round your shoulders, and pull your knees into your body, spreading them apart – this allows all your muscles to work. Steady pushes help bring your baby down easier and quicker through the birth canal. Be sure you completely relax and rest between each contraction.

The location of your baby's head as it moves through your pelvis (called descent) is reported in a number called a station. If the baby's head has not started its descent, the station is described at minus three (-3). When your baby's head is at the zero station, it is at the middle of the birth canal and is said to be engaged in the pelvis. The station of your baby helps indicate the progress of the second stage of labor.

When your baby is born, your healthcare provider will hold the baby with his or her head lowered to prevent amniotic fluid, mucus and blood from getting into the baby's lungs. The baby's mouth and nose may be suctioned with a small bulb syringe to remove any additional fluid. Your provider will place the baby on your stomach and shortly after, the umbilical cord will be cut.

**Third Stage** - The third stage of labor begins after the baby is born and ends when the placenta separates from the wall of the uterus and is passed through the vagina. This stage is often called delivery of the "afterbirth" and is the shortest stage of labor. It may last from a few minutes to 30 minutes. You will feel contractions but they will be less painful. If you had an episiotomy or small tear, it will be stitched during this stage of labor.

If you have any further questions regarding labor and birth, please discuss them with your healthcare provider at your prenatal visits.

## Frequently Asked Questions about Labor

### When does labor begin?

Labor begins when the cervix begins to open (dilate) and thin (called effacement). The muscles of the uterus tighten (contract) at regular intervals. During contractions, the abdomen becomes hard. Between contractions, the uterus relaxes and the abdomen becomes soft.

### How will I know if I'm in labor?

Some women experience very distinct signs of labor, while others don't. No one knows what causes labor to start, but several hormonal and physical changes may indicate the beginning of labor. These changes include:

*Lightening* - The process of your baby settling or lowering into your pelvis is called lightening. Lightening can happen a few weeks or a few hours before labor. Because the uterus rests on the bladder more after lightening, you may feel the need to urinate more frequently.

*Mucus Plug* - The mucus plug accumulates at the cervix during pregnancy. When the cervix begins to open wider, the mucus is discharged into the vagina and may be clear, pink or slightly bloody. Labor may begin soon after the mucus plug is discharged or may begin one to two weeks later.

### *What are contractions?*

Labor is characterized by contractions, the tightening and relaxing of the uterine muscle, that come at regular intervals and increase in frequency (how often contractions occur), duration (how long contractions last) and intensity (how strong the contractions are). As time progresses, the contractions come at closer intervals.

Labor contractions cause discomfort or a dull ache in your back and lower abdomen, along with pressure in the pelvis. Some women describe contractions as strong menstrual cramps. You may have a small amount of bleeding from your vagina. Labor contractions are not stopped by changing your position or relaxing. Although the contractions may be uncomfortable, you will be able to relax in between contractions.

This part of the first stage of labor (called the Latent Phase) is best experienced in the comfort of your home. Keep in telephone contact with your healthcare provider to let him/her know of your progress. He/she will advise you on what is best to eat and drink at this time. Fluids are very important to consume in early labor to prevent dehydration.

---

### Coping with Contractions

- Try to distract yourself – take a walk, go shopping, watch a movie.
- Soak in a warm tub or take a warm shower. Allow the showerhead water to pulsate on your lower back as it may help with the lower back discomfort.
- Try to sleep if it is in the evening. You need to store up your energy for labor.

---

### *How do I time my contractions?*

At the beginning of one contraction and again at the beginning of the next contraction, write down the time. The time between contractions includes the length or duration of the contraction and the minutes in between the contractions (called the interval).

Mild contractions generally begin 15 to 20 minutes apart and last 45 to 60 seconds. The contractions become more regular until they are less than five minutes apart. Active labor is usually characterized by strong contractions that last 60 to 90 seconds and experienced three to five minutes apart. Another indication that you are progressing is when you are unable to talk through a contraction and must concentrate on breathing. Have your birth plan handy. If you planned to deliver your baby in a hospital or medical center, now is the time you should go there.

### What happens when my water breaks?

The rupture of the amniotic membrane (the fluid-filled sac that surrounds your baby during pregnancy) is also referred to as your "bag of water breaking." The rupture of the amniotic membrane may feel either like a sudden gush of fluid or a trickle of fluid that leaks steadily. The fluid is usually odorless and may look clear or straw-colored.

If your "water breaks," notify your healthcare provider. Tell your provider what time your bag of water broke, how much fluid was released and what the fluid looked like. Labor may or may not start soon after your bag of water breaks.

It is also common to be in labor without your water breaking. Actually, only thirty percent of women experience their water breaking prior to the start of labor.

### What is effacement and dilation of the cervix?

Your cervix gets shorter and thins out in order to stretch and open around your baby's head. The shortening and thinning of the cervix is called effacement and is measured in percentages from 0 to 100 percent. The stretching and opening of your cervix is called dilation and is measured from 1 to 10 centimeters.

Effacement and dilation are a direct result of effective uterine contractions. Progress in labor is measured by how much the cervix has opened and thinned to allow your baby to pass through the vagina.

### When should I call my healthcare provider or go to the hospital?

Call your provider during early labor, when you have a question or concern, or if you are unsure if you are in true labor or experiencing false labor. Also call:
- If you think your water has broken (if there is a sudden gush of fluid or a trickle of fluid that leaks steadily).
- If you are bleeding (more than spotting).

- When your contractions are very uncomfortable and have been coming every five minutes for an hour.

Your healthcare provider will give you specific guidelines about when you should get ready to come to the hospital.

## What Should I bring to the Hospital?

We recommend packing your bag ahead of time (two to four weeks before your due date), so you have one less thing to worry about as you prepare to come to the hospital. Since your hospital stay will be short, try to bring just what you need. Do not bring any medications, valuable jewelry, credit cards or large amounts of cash. We suggest packing:

*Mom's Suitcase:*
- Personal toiletries – toothbrush, toothpaste, hair care products, skin care products
- Glasses or contacts and supplies (if appropriate)
- One or two night gowns (optional – hospital gowns are provided) and a robe
- Slippers, socks
- Underwear (3 or 4 pairs, cotton) and nursing bras
- List of names and phone numbers of family and friends you'll want to call to share your news
- A book or magazine, a deck of cards
- Comfortable clothes to go home in
- (Optional) Your camera, camcorder, or tape recorder (with cassette tapes or blank tapes, spare batteries and chargers); iPod with your favorite music

*Baby's Bag:*
- Undershirt
- Socks
- Receiving blanket
- Clothes to go home in (depending on the weather, you may need to include a hat, sweater, or snowsuit)
- Infant car seat

*Note*: Everything your baby needs for his or her stay in the hospital will be provided, including diapers.

Since your partner or support person will be staying in the hospital with you, he or she should bring personal toiletries, comfortable clothes for sleeping, slippers, socks and a change of clothes. He or she may want to bring some money to buy food in the cafeteria.

## What Happens When I Get to the Hospital?

Expectant mothers are seen on the Labor and Delivery Unit for admission to the hospital or for testing. You will be shown to your labor, delivery and recovery room (LDR) at this time. (You may have already toured the hospital at a previous point in time.)

You may be asked to wear a hospital gown or if you like, you can wear your own comfortable, loose-fitting clothing.

Your pulse, blood pressure and temperature will be checked. A monitor will be placed on your abdomen for a short time to check for uterine contractions and assess the baby's heart rate. Your healthcare provider will also examine your cervix to determine how far labor has progressed.

A saline lock may be placed into a vein in your arm for immediate access to deliver fluids and medications if necessary.

It sounds overwhelming and it can be if you aren't warned about what happens. If you know, as we've outlined here, then you can remain calm and know that everything is progressing just as it should.

## Types of Births

**Vaginal birth** is the most common and safest type of childbirth. In certain circumstances, forceps (instruments resembling large spoons) may be used to cup your baby's head and help guide the baby through the birth canal while you are pushing. This is performed by your healthcare provider. Vacuum-assisted delivery is another way to assist birth and is similar to forceps delivery. In vacuum-assisted delivery, a plastic cup is applied to the baby's head by suction and your healthcare provider gently pulls the baby from the birth canal while you aid with your pushing efforts. If your healthcare provider is a nurse-midwife, her collaborating physician will be the individual performing the vacuum-assisted and/or forceps-assisted delivery. Ask questions regarding a vacuum-assisted and forceps-assisted birth during your prenatal visits and the circumstances that would necessitate that type of intervention.

**Cesarean section** is sometimes necessary for the safest outcome for you and your baby. A cesarean birth may be necessary if one of the following complications is present:

- Your baby is not in the head-down position, or is in an abnormal position for a vaginal birth, such as breech (buttocks coming first); transverse (side ways), etc.
- Your baby is too large to pass through the pelvis.
- Your baby is in distress. This is indicated by the baby's heart rate showing it is not getting enough oxygen by slowing down its rate.
- Your placenta is covering the opening to the cervix (placenta previa).
- Your placenta separates from the wall of your uterus before the baby is born (abruption of placenta).
- You have active outbreak of the herpes virus in or near the vagina near the time of birth.
- Labor is not progressing adequately.

Talk to your healthcare provider during your prenatal visits to discuss what options are available to you if you would need to have a cesarean section.

---

### Questions to Review with your Healthcare Provider

- What cesarean procedure you and the hospital use routinely?
- Do you use a two-layer closure on your uterus for possibility of having a future vaginal birth?
- Is my spouse/partner (or support person) allowed in the operating and recovery rooms with me?
- Do I have the option to breastfeed in the operating room or in the recovery room?

---

A cesarean birth can be a couple-centered experience if you are prepared for what to expect during that situation. It is not a sign of failure on your part if you cannot achieve a vaginal birth if that was your original intention. Being prepared and knowing what to expect will make the experience easier for both you and your partner.

The old saying "once a cesarean, always a cesarean" is just that: an old saying. Frequently, it is safe to birth your next baby vaginally. However, this should be discussed with your healthcare provider. They will review your operative report to determine your type of uterine scar to determine if you are a good candidate for a VBAC (vaginal birth after cesarean section).

A cesarean section is major abdominal surgery, so recovery will be the same as any other major surgery. Rest is vital for a successful recovery from cesarean birth. Be sure to follow your going-home instructions and recruit help at home while you are recovering. Staying in contact with your healthcare provider during your postpartum/post-operative recovery is a keystone of a successful postpartum course.

# Conclusion

Congratulations on your birth and becoming a mom! You should view your labor and birth as a rite of passage into a new and exciting role! The first few weeks after your baby's birth are to be cherished. Times of transition require special attention so people can move confidently into their new roles.

# Physiological Changes in the Postpartum Period

There are many changes, physically, emotionally, and psychologically that occur over the next two months. Your body will experience numerous changes, some of which continue for several weeks during your postpartum period. Like pregnancy, postpartum changes are different for every woman.

Simply, the postpartum period is the time from the delivery of the placenta and membranes to the return of your reproductive tract to its non-pregnant condition. Please note that we said non-pregnant condition, not pre-pregnant condition. The pre-pregnant condition of your reproductive organs is gone forever – their shape and size will remain enlarged, but this is something you will not be aware of from the outside of your body. This is why it is critical to be patient as you body heals.

## General Physiological Changes

A woman in labor goes through a tremendous amount of stress and strain; and it takes some time for her general condition to return to a normal state again.

**Pulse Rate:** Your pulse rate normally rises during the course of labor. It continues to be unpredictable in the first two days after your baby's birth, and then returns to normal by the third day. However, any pulse rate more than 100 beats per minute at any time should be investigated for fever or excessive blood loss.

**Temperature:** Your temperature often becomes sub-normal after birth. This low temperature can cause you to shiver in an attempt to raise your body temperature again. It comes back to normal within 24 hours. On the third day, there may be a slight rise in your temperature because of the let down reflex of milk with a consequent mild engorgement of your breasts.

**Changes in the blood:** Immediately after your birth there is a slight decrease in your total blood volume due to dehydration and blood loss. This returns to normal within seven days. Your hemoglobin stabilizes by the fifth day. WBC count (white blood cell) which increases during pregnancy comes back to normal in one week. Platelet count and fibrinogen level however increases at around the 4th to the 10th day after birth and then comes back to normal in about another two weeks.

**Urinary Tract:** The urinary tract is placed under a lot of stress during labor. The bladder wall becomes edematous and swollen, and the muscles of the urethra become loose and flabby due to stretching during birth. Pressure from the baby's head tends to decrease the strength of your bladder and urethra. As a result, you may have some difficulty in passing urine for the first 24 hours after your birth. But the muscle tone is regained in one to two days. There is an increased tendency to pass urine in the first two days to eliminate water retained during pregnancy.

**Gastro-intestinal tract:** There may be increased thirst during the first few days after birth since there is increased fluid loss in the lochia, urine and also in sweating. Constipation can occur as a result of dehydration. General pain in the vaginal and perineal areas can also contribute to constipation.

**Weight Loss:** A weight loss of about 10.2 pounds takes place at the time of the birth of your baby, placenta, membranes and amniotic fluid. A further loss of about 7.6 pounds takes place during the puerperium, the medical term for the time immediately following delivery, due to the elimination of water and decreased size of the uterus.

So, in a woman with a standard weight gain of 25.4 pounds during pregnancy, there is a weight loss of 17.8 pounds after birth. She will thus have a net weight gain of 7.6 pounds due to pregnancy.

## *Vaginal Bleeding after Birth*

Vaginal discharge after birth is called lochia. It is a combination of the old uterine lining and blood. The lochia usually changes from bright red, to pink, to brownish to white in color over the course of several weeks. Lochia is not your period. You will experience lochia whether you have a vaginal birth or a cesarean birth. Vaginal bleeding after a cesarean will usually be less than after a vaginal birth.

It is very common for your bleeding to start and stop and to have clots. Passing blood clots in lochia is normal as long as they gradually become less frequent, become smaller and are not accompanied by heavy bleeding or cramping. Your bleeding (lochia) will be heavy at first and will decrease over time.

If your lochia has decreased substantially and then increases again and turns bright red, this is an indication that you are doing too much physically. Decrease your physical activity, as it is a sign for you to slow down and rest more. Bleeding can also increase after breastfeeding or after lying down.

*Types of Lochia*

**Lochia Rubra** occurs in the first three to four days after childbirth. It is reddish in color and is made up of mainly blood, bits of fetal membranes, decidua (uterine lining), meconium (the earliest stools of an infant) and cervical discharge.

**Lochia Serosa** gradually changes color to brown and then yellow over a period of about one week. It is called lochia serosa at this stage. The lochia serosa contains fewer red blood cells but more white blood cells, wound discharge from the placental and other sites, and mucus from the cervix.

**Lochia Alba** is a whitish, turbid fluid which drains from the vagina for about another one to two weeks. It mainly consists of decidual cells, mucus, white blood cells, and epithelial cells.

The lochia has a characteristic 'fishy' odor, which is easily recognizable. But in puerperal or postpartum infections, there may be a foul smell due to the presence of bacteria and pus in the discharge.

---

**Do Not Use Tampons**

Use sanitary pads instead of tampons until you have your first menstrual period after birth or until your healthcare provider advises otherwise.

---

## Involution of the Uterus

The uterus, which weighs about 900 grams at the end of labor, weighs only about 60 grams at the end of the postpartum period, six weeks after childbirth.

Immediately after your birth, the uterus becomes a firm, immobile structure located just above your pubic bone. It is about 20 cm in length and, in a woman of average height, will reach up to the umbilicus (navel or belly button). It is slightly tender when palpated.

The uterus begins to return to its non-pregnancy size immediately after birth. It shrinks from about the size of a basketball during pregnancy, to the size of a grapefruit right after birth and, finally, to the size of a small pear by six weeks after birth. Your uterus will shrink to your navel at first and gradually descend back into your pelvis over a period of 10-14 days. This rapid decrease in the size is reflected in the changing location of the uterus as it descends out of the abdomen and again returns to being a pelvic organ. The broad and round ligaments of the uterus which stretched to accommodate the uterus during its increase in size are now lax as a result of the extreme stretching, but by the end of six weeks will regain their non-pregnant length and tension.

While your uterus is going through the process of involution, you may experience mild to moderate contractions called after-pains. After-pains are lower abdominal colicky pains due to irregular uterine spasms. If the uterus is empty of any blood clots or retained placenta bits, supportive treatment in the form of pain relieving medicines and counseling is all that is required. After-pains can be very uncomfortable, but they are weaker than labor contractions and will become milder over the next few days. The contractions may feel more intense while you are breastfeeding because your baby's sucking triggers the release of your natural oxytocin that causes your uterus to contract. Your after-pains will be more painful with each subsequent birth because the uterus has to work harder to get back to its normal non-pregnant state.

The size of the uterus decreases at the rate of one-half inch per 24 hours in the first 14 days of the postpartum period. It regains its non-pregnancy size at the end of six weeks.

## *Involution of the Cervix*

The cervix involutes more slowly than the uterus. Immediately after the birth of your baby, it is a loose opening with irregular edges. But by the end of the first week, it becomes more clearly defined, regaining its canal like structure. Its opening in the vagina now is much smaller and can admit only the tip of the finger. While the internal os, which is the opening of the cervix near the uterus involutes completely, the external os, which is the outer opening of the cervix in the vagina, never regains its pre-pregnant state.

# *Vagina and Perineum*

Immediately post birth, your vagina remains quite stretched, may have some bruising and edema, and may gape open at the introitus (vaginal opening). Your vagina will always be a little larger than it was prior to your first childbirth. Perineal muscle tightening exercises (Kegel exercises) will restore its tone and enable deliberate tightening of the vagina to a considerable degree. This can be accomplished by the end of six weeks with daily practice.

Involution of the vagina: The vagina involutes more slowly than the uterus. The normal rugosity (wrinkles) of the vaginal walls reappears about the third week of the postpartum period. But the size and elasticity of the tissues never regain the pre-pregnancy state.

Your perineum may be sore and slightly swollen after birth. If you had a tear (laceration) or an episiotomy, your perineum will be tender (see below). The swelling does decrease in a few days. Any increased pain or increased swelling should be reported to your healthcare provider.

*For your comfort:*
- Wash hands before and after changing pads, before using a peri bottle, etc.
- Always wipe from front to back (toward your rectum) after bowel movements and urination.
- Wash your perineum daily with mild soap and water during your shower or bath. Avoid any perfumed body washes or soaps. Avoid deodorant body soaps.
- Change peri pads when necessary and after going to the restroom.

---

### Use of the Peri Bottle

1. Fill the bottle with plain warm water.
2. Sit on the toilet.
3. Remove soiled peri pad.
4. Squeeze bottle to rinse perineum.
5. Pat dry with soft tissue, from the front to the back (toward your rectum) or just let air dry.
6. Put on a clean peri pad each time you use the bathroom.

---

## *Lacerations, Abrasions & Episiotomy*

If you had an episiotomy or a laceration that was repaired, the stitches will dissolve in about two weeks and do not need to be removed. The skin heals in about two to three weeks. You may see small pieces of the stitches in your underwear as your episiotomy or laceration heals. This is normal and no cause for concern.

Immediately after birth and whenever swelling is present use an ice pack for comfort for the first 24 hours postpartum. You may also use a portable sitz bath or sit in a shallow amount of warm bath water. Repeat three to four times per day for about 10 minutes, until the swelling has gone. Alternating heat and cold may be helpful.

Perineal pain usually improves daily. Take a mild pain reliever (such as acetaminophen or ibuprofen) if needed. Many women find that sitting on a hard surface is usually more comfortable if they squeeze their buttocks together and hold the contraction while sitting down. Keep the perineum dry and wear cotton underwear. Apply witch-hazel compresses to help reduce discomfort. You can also use a foam cushion to sit on if sitting is painful. Begin Kegel exercises as soon as possible. You will appreciate its effects as you progress through your postpartum period.

Caring for your perineum becomes even more important if you had a more extensive perineal tear (into the anus or rectum). Most women find frequent sitz baths (four to five times per day) comforting and healing. Squirt warm water from your peri bottle onto the area where you urinate to prevent stinging and help keep the area clean. This is essential if you have stitches.

Do not get too active too soon. Avoid lifting anything heavier than your baby and don't overdo the stair climbing!

Keep your stool soft with an OTC (over-the-counter) stool softener and be sure to increase your fiber, fresh fruits and raw veggies. A small juice glass size of cold prune juice before bed every night is also beneficial. You can also consume fresh prunes on a daily basis. Of course, continue to drink plenty of water!

If you notice a foul odor or have trouble controlling your stool, call your healthcare provider immediately.

## *Breasts*

The nipple and areola (the dark area around the nipple) enlarge and darken during pregnancy. This may help your baby latch on by providing a clear "target." Each nipple has 15 to 20 openings for milk to flow.

The small bumps on the areola are called Montgomery glands. They produce natural oil that cleans, lubricates, and protects the nipple during pregnancy and breastfeeding. This oil contains an enzyme that kills bacteria and makes breast creams unnecessary. You should use only water to clean your breasts. Soaps, lotions or alcohol might remove this protective oil.

When your baby nurses, the action of baby's jaw and tongue pressing down on the milk sinuses creates suction. This causes the milk to flow out of your breast and into your baby's mouth.

While you were pregnant, your body was preparing a very special blend of nutrients to meet your baby's needs. Colostrum (early breast milk) is the perfect starter food for your baby! This yellowish, creamy substance is found in the breasts during pregnancy and for a few days after birth. Your colostrum provides all the nutrition your baby will need right after birth. The quantity available of this "liquid gold" is close to the capacity of the newborn's stomach. It also provides important protection against bacteria and viruses.

Colostrum acts as natural laxative (something that makes it easier to have bowel movements) to help clear the meconium (the dark sticky stool that is made while the baby is in the uterus) from your baby's intestines. Meconium contains bilirubin, the substance that causes newborn jaundice. Colostrum in frequent doses helps eliminate bilirubin from the body, which may lessen or decrease the severity of newborn jaundice. Colostrum also acts as a seal to the newborn's intestines, preventing invasion of bacteria and provides the newborn with high levels of antibodies from you. Colostrum is the ideal nutrient for the first few days of your baby's life, and is high in protein and low in sugar and fat, making it easier to digest. The protein content is three times higher than mature milk, because it is rich in the antibodies being passed from the mother.

The amount of breast milk you make will increase over the first few days after birth. Breast milk is the perfect balance of water and nutrients containing fats, sugars, proteins, minerals, vitamins, antibodies and enzymes. It is also designed to promote brain and body growth. As your baby grows older, your milk changes to meet your baby's nutritional needs. Breastfeeding also allows you and your baby to bond in a way that cannot be matched by bottle feeding. Breastfeeding success has nothing to do with the size of your breasts or nipples. Breast size is an inherited trait and determined by the number of fat cells you have. Your breasts will enlarge with pregnancy and with breastfeeding. Breastfeeding is a supply-and-demand process. Therefore, the more you nurse, the more milk you produce!

When your milk supply increases, around 48 to 72 hours after birth, your breasts may become firm and a little tender. Fullness in your breasts occurs naturally from an increase in blood flow. This prepares your breasts for increased milk production. If you are breastfeeding, nursing often will help keep your breasts soft and prevent engorgement.

If you want to breastfeed but are experiencing difficulty doing so, seek help from your healthcare provider. Many hospitals often have trained professionals that can help with this specifically, and can be scheduled to come into your room to coach you. There are also breastfeeding specialists who will come to your home to help. If breastfeeding is just not working out, ask your healthcare provider about what formulas they recommend as best for your baby.

If you are not breastfeeding, a snug-fitting bra like a sports bra or towels wrapped tightly around both breasts will help minimize breast engorgement. If your breasts become painful, avoid nipple stimulation and milk expression; when showering, do not let water stimulate breasts; avoid warm water directly on your breasts as this may increase milk production.

---

### Soothing Engorged Breasts

If engorgement is really painful, bend over a pan of warm water and put your breasts into the water. After a minute or so, milk will flow without stimulating your breasts. Apply ice packs to decrease the swelling and consider taking a mild pain reliever. You can also place fresh cabbage leaves in the cups of your bra for comfort.

---

## *Hemorrhoids*

Many women develop hemorrhoids during pregnancy and after giving birth. Hemorrhoids are varicose veins of the rectum caused by the weight and pressure of your baby and from the force of pushing. Hemorrhoid pain may be relieved with ice packs, ice-cold pads containing Witch Hazel, or your healthcare provider may suggest other creams or suppositories.

As mentioned above, reduce the risk of constipation by eating fruits, vegetables and whole grains and drinking lots of fluids. Prunes and bran are helpful remedies if you have a tendency toward constipation. You may also be prescribed a stool softener. Contact your healthcare provider for recommendations. Hemorrhoids will eventually shrink and become less uncomfortable.

## *Bladder*

It may be slightly uncomfortable to urinate for a few days after your baby's birth. Pain or burning when you urinate, or the urge to urinate frequently, may indicate a bladder infection and should be reported to your healthcare provider.

*Helpful hints to avoid a bladder infection:*
- Drink plenty of water.
- If you are having trouble urinating, try turning on the faucet when you are on the toilet. The sound of running water may help you urinate.
- Pour a peri bottle filled with warm water over your perineum as you sit on the toilet.
- Urinating often to empty your bladder may decrease your chance of bladder infection. It also helps decrease cramping.
- Urinate while using a warm sitz bath or in the shower.

## *Bowels*

Your bowel movements may be delayed until three or four days after childbirth because of the lack of food during labor and discomfort from hemorrhoids or any lacerations or episiotomy. Do not hold back a bowel movement, even if it is uncomfortable. Ask your healthcare provider about over-the-counter stool softeners if you have problems.

*Helpful hints to avoid constipation:*
- Eat a high-fiber diet (fresh fruits and vegetables, whole grains, etc.).
- Drink plenty of fluids.
- Walk as much as is comfortable.
- Exercise as your healthcare provider recommends.

# Menstruation

Your menstrual period may not resume while you are breastfeeding. If it does, it should not interfere with breastfeeding but may slightly decrease the amount of breast milk available. Drink lots of fluids often, and your milk supply will stabilize.

The return of the first menstrual period after the birth of your baby is variable and depends to a great extent on whether you are breastfeeding. If bottle-feeding, your period may return within four to twelve weeks. By the end of the 12th week, almost 80% of all women who do not breastfeed have their first menstrual period.

Your first period may be heavier than normal. There may be clots, and the bleeding may start and stop. Ovulation returns approximately four weeks after giving birth unless you are breastfeeding. In women who do not breastfeed, ovulation returns four weeks after birth and menstruation returns after six weeks in about 40% of all women. By the end of the 12th week, almost 80% of all women who do not breastfeed have got their first menstrual period.

In women who breastfeed, menstruation returns about six to seven months after childbirth. But this, too, depends on how long the woman breastfed her baby exclusively without any supplementary feeds.

According to most pediatricians, babies need to be exclusively breastfed for the first six months of life. In such a case, menstruation may return later than six to seven months.

# Fatigue

Even mothers in top physical condition prior to birth may feel a great deal of fatigue in the early recovery period. Feeling continually tired might last weeks or even months. Recognize that your body has been through a major physical process and that you need to allow yourself enough recovery time.

*Tips for coping with fatigue:*

- Remain in your bathrobe or lounge wear for the first week at home and rest whenever possible. New babies tend to be more awake at night than during the day for the first three weeks, so be prepared to rest when your baby sleeps.
- Let others help with household chores, such as laundry, cooking, shopping, cleaning, etc. When friends offer to help, let them!
- If possible, arrange to have your partner take one to two weeks off after the baby arrives.
- If possible, hire outside help for a few hours during the first weeks, even if your partner will be off work and helping. You will both need some time to adjust and be with the baby.
- If you have an answering machine or voice mail, you may wish to leave a message stating that you are resting and will call when you have the time to talk. Consider renting or borrowing an answering machine if you do not have one.
- Make life as simple as possible by using paper plates, take-out food and delivery services. Take it easy!
- Limit the amount of visitors the first couple of weeks. This is not the time to feel you have to play hostess and entertain.
- Review your diet to be sure you have enough protein and iron in your diet. For more information on iron, ask your healthcare provider about iron supplements

## *Additional Physical Changes*

Once you give birth, there is a large change in the amount of certain hormones in your body. These changes can affect the amount of fluid in your body and can cause some common physical changes including:

- Retention of fluid/swelling
- Initial hair loss (your hair will come in again later)
- Hot flashes
- Night sweats
- Dry skin
- Mood swings
- Increased urination
- Vaginal dryness

It is important to understand that it took nine months for your body to go through all of the changes that it did during pregnancy, and many people believe you should give yourself at least nine months to recover fully from the changes that occur during pregnancy.

# Emotional Changes

In addition to the physiological changes you will experience after giving birth, often it takes time for a woman's emotional and mental balance to return to normal.

## *Postpartum Depression*

"Why do I feel sad and detached? I am so overwhelmed and anxious about everything. Isn't this supposed to be one of the happiest times in my life? Then why don't I feel happy? How am I supposed to take care of my baby when I don't have the energy to even take a shower? Gosh, to be honest, I don't even have the energy or desire to get out of bed..."

Most people have heard of this term but might have a difficult time explaining how to recognize it. If you are one of those who have suffered from it, you will never forget how it felt...

Many women right after giving birth suffer from some level of anxiety or sadness, irritability and mood swings, trouble with sleeping and low appetite, and many cry easily. Statistics show as many as 80% of women experience some mood disturbances after pregnancy. It can start as soon as 24 hours after giving birth but is usually three to four days after. This is what many call the "baby blues." You can still be experiencing the baby blues even if this isn't your first child and you have never had any concerns before.

### What causes the baby blues?

Your body is going through so many changes now. Your hormone levels are dropping, your body is making milk for breastfeeding and you are physically (and mentally) trying to adjust to all that a mother of a newborn deals with. It's no wonder you feel anxious and overwhelmed. The baby blues are perfectly understandable. Moms have to remember it isn't something they can control and shouldn't blame themselves. The baby blues are considered by many as a normal part of motherhood. For most, the baby blues last from a few days up to a little more than a week. If these feelings continue, or seem to get worse, it might be more than just the baby blues.

### What is postpartum depression?

In the beginning postpartum depression can look like just the baby blues. The length and severity of the symptoms are what separates the two. About 10% of new mothers experience postpartum depression. The exact cause isn't known, but as with the baby blues, sudden hormonal changes are believed to be part of the cause of postpartum depression. One theory is the levels of estrogen and progesterone that have increased during pregnancy drop suddenly after delivery and produce chemical changes in the brain. Researchers think the big change in hormone levels is what may lead to depression in some.

Postpartum depression usually sets in soon after childbirth and develops gradually over a period of several months. It is important to note postpartum depression can come on suddenly, months even after delivery, and the first signs don't appear until then. If depressive symptoms appear within six months of having a baby, postpartum depression should be considered. It is important to speak with your health care provider if you feel it might be more than just the baby blues. Postpartum depression needs to be treated and won't disappear on its own.

### What are the signs of postpartum depression?
- Lack of interest in your baby
- Lack of energy and motivation
- Feelings of guilt and worthlessness
- Loss of pleasure in things that use to bring pleasure
- Negative feelings toward your baby
- Worrying about hurting yourself or your baby
- Changes in appetite or weight
- Sleeping more or less than usual
- Recurrent thoughts of death or suicide

## *Mood Boosting Techniques*

Whether it is the baby blues or depression, here are a few suggestions that can help:

**Exercising** – For some people exercise works as well as antidepressants and you will look better, sleep better, and hopefully feel less depressed. A helpful tip is to exercise with others for support.

**Continuing to eat a healthy diet** – Build around fruits and vegetables, and limit unhealthy fat and sugars. Incorporate flaxseeds, nuts and dark green vegetables for a great foundation.

**Supplementation** – B complex vitamins B6, B-12 and folic acid along with omega-3 fatty acids have been shown to ease mood changes and depression symptoms. For example B6 is essential for the body's production of serotonin, which most antidepressant drugs are designed to elevate.

**Healthy carbohydrates** – Eaten alone without protein raises the levels of serotonin. Good options are baked sweet potatoes, whole wheat pasta and healthy crackers.

**Be careful with coffee** – Caffeine can make you jittery and anxious all by itself so it might be a good time to limit intake.

**Get lots of sunshine and fresh air** – Sunlight has been shown to benefit depression.

**Do something that gives you pleasure** – Take time to do the things you enjoy because you are worth it!

**Need to rest and relax your mind** – Stress and anxiety can make depression symptoms worse. This can be a great time to take that yoga class or a good time to learn the art of meditation.

**Continue to engage with your social network as much as possible** – Engage with those around you on a regular basis. You have a new role as Mom of a little one but it is important to keep our connections with others strong as well.

**Sleep is SO important** – I am sure you are asking, "What is sleep?" You always hear "sleep when your baby sleeps" but it is so true. Getting enough rest and establishing good sleeping habits for you (and your baby) will help you feel better both mentally and physically.

**Avoid Alcohol & Drugs** – They can make depression and anxiety worse and can prevent recovery.

**Seeking treatment when needed is very important** – Depression is a serious illness. Medical treatment and counseling can be a very important component to recovery and a healthy life. Make sure you talk with your healthcare provider to help you get in touch with those in your area who are trained to help.

---

**Call Your Healthcare Provider if You Experience Any of the Following**

- You feel so overwhelmed you can't perform tasks you need to
- Your symptoms of depression seem to get more and more intense
- You are unable to care for yourself or your baby
- You have thoughts of harming yourself or your baby

---

It is important to understand postpartum depression can begin anytime within the first year after childbirth.

# Months 0-2

Giving birth is one of the most incredible moments in your life. You spent the last nine months going through lots of physical changes (and some emotional changes too) to welcome that beautiful baby in your arms. You feel like this should be the end of your body's long journey and now you can both physically and emotionally get back to normal…right? Even if your labor was uneventful and easy it will take some time to feel like yourself again. Even if you were blessed with great genes, you won't get there overnight.

Many mothers will go through dramatic changes both emotionally and physically after the birth process. Some of the psychological issues prevalent in new mothers are depression, excessive emotional reactions such as crying easily, self-esteem issues and frequent mood changes.

Another thing you might notice is how tired you are. After the birth, it is not unusual for women to feel like they just ran a marathon. All mothers feel some level of fatigue in the early recovery period. This tired feeling may last for quite some time. Your body is telling you it needs time to recover and it's important to listen to it. The six-week postnatal period is extremely important for supporting new moms back to health.

## Give Your Body Plenty of Time to Heal!

What most of us don't understand is that a woman's body can take as long to recover as pregnancy itself. Women who give birth go through a complete physical and emotional change and will require extra support for quite some time. The recovery time will depend on how complicated your birth was and whether you had a cesarean section.

New moms need to allow themselves time to recover physically and mentally, and re-adjust after giving birth. Moms need to remember THEY are just as important as their babies in the post birth recovery process. A happy and healthy mom will make for a happy and healthy baby.

Between sleep deprivation and the needs of the new baby, many moms wonder how they can find the time or the energy to take care of themselves. Some mothers can struggle with guilt for taking time for them and still feeling committed to taking care of their family. Moms need to understand it is ok to want (and need) time for her. The more moms can take care of themselves, the quicker their recovery.

## Pregnancy & Birth Takes an Emotional Toll as Well!

Pregnancy and birth can wreak havoc on a woman's emotions! Your hormone levels are continuously fluctuating through pregnancy and well beyond your birth. You can understand how this can lead to feelings of mental exhaustion, anxiety, sadness and for some, depression. Most of the time these feelings will subside once your hormones level out and your body has time to recover.

The key to addressing any psychological effects of hormonal fluctuations is to recognize the changes that are occurring are normal. With adequate support most mothers will readjust from pregnancy and birth very well on an emotional basis, if they know what to expect and how to deal with it ahead of time.

## What are Good First Steps?

Ask for help if possible! Most of your time will be spent caring for you and your baby. You shouldn't be stressing about the household chores. If it's possible, enlist the help of your spouse, family or even friends to help maintain the house and cook meals. Once you are feeling better you can coordinate something special for them.

**Exercise** – Exercise will help you mentally and physically regain your strength and relieve some of the stress. Try to do something light and easy everyday to start with. Don't over exercise. Take a short walk with your baby in the stroller. Most gyms offer childcare facilities, so check your local gym or find one close by that offers this. Gyms are a great way to get a little time for yourself to do something good for your mind and your body.

**Eating Healthy** – This isn't the time for drastic dieting, especially if you are breastfeeding, it is the time to make sure you are eating healthy! Just as you did when you were pregnant, ensure you're not eating empty calories.

**Treat yourself** – Allow yourself time for some serious pampering. Find time for that much needed massage or spa day. Your body will thank you!

**Stay positive** – Studies show that a positive attitude after childbirth is associated with a faster recovery process, so try to stay as positive as possible.

**Sleep** - Try to get as much sleep as you can. For new moms sleep can be scarce and inconsistent, but very important for maintaining health and well-being.

---

### Mom-to-Mom Tip: Sleep When Your Baby Sleeps!

You will be very tempted to use this time to catch up while your baby sleeps but for your emotional and physical well-being, try to sleep when you baby sleeps. If you can't do this every time, strive to do it half or three-fourths of the time. If you are breastfeeding it is very important to get as much sleep as possible to ensure adequate milk supply to feed your baby.

Get your spouse or partner involved. You will need to wake up three to four times a night to feed your newborn. Get your partner involved in the feeding. You can pump your breast milk and let you partner feed the baby and change the diaper if needed while you rest.

To keep track of your baby's sleep cycle, visit our website at www.9monthsin9monthsout.com to download a sleep chart. This will help you track your baby's sleeping patterns and help you figure out the best time to get your sleep in as well.

---

# Maternal & Infant Nutrition

Sure, you may be feeling, well, HUGE after having your baby, but that doesn't mean now is the time to try out a crazy fad diet. What your body needs is proper nutrition. Women are designed to lose baby weight after having a baby, but after years of working with moms postpartum, and doing it ourselves, we know that losing baby weight is sometimes the hardest weight to lose. But it doesn't have to be. It took nine months to gain the weight, so you need to give yourself *at least nine months* to take it all off. (Okay, it might happen faster than that, or more slowly, but the key is giving yourself a fair amount of time to do it).

A pregnant body undergoes many changes during pregnancy, especially with the birth of your baby. Moms need time to heal and recover and a healthy nutritional foundation promotes more complete healing. The weight gained throughout pregnancy helps build stores for recovery and breastfeeding. Postnatal nutrition is usually broken down into two specific categories: Mom's nutritional needs and Baby's nutritional needs.

In our book we will primarily focus on "Mom's" needs! And whether you breastfeed or bottle feed, all moms need a healthy diet full of fruits, vegetables, lean protein, whole grains and vitamins and minerals. Along with balanced meals, breastfeeding mothers should increase fluids. Many mothers find they become very thirsty while the baby is nursing. Water, milk, and fruit juices (but watch sugar content) are excellent choices. It is helpful to keep a pitcher of water and even some healthy snacks beside your bed or breastfeeding chair.

A goal of losing one to two pounds a week is the maximum recommended in order to keep up your strength and bone density. Milk production requires an extra 500 calories/day and healthcare providers recommend that women who nurse maintain an extra five to ten pounds. This is primarily due to maintaining healthy levels of estrogen, which will make you feel a little softer, but think health of the baby here. Although early milk production draws on weight gained during pregnancy, it is important to consume enough calories to keep up your energy level during this time of healing and change. You should not, however, consume more calories than necessary.

If something is lacking in Mom's current diet, Mom's body will dip into her reserves of nutrients to keep breast milk nutrient-dense. However, you are going to need your body to be healthy for a long time to take care of your growing child, so don't short-change yourself!

Be assured that the composition of nutrients in human milk is consistent. A nutrition shortage for mom is more likely to reduce the quantity of milk than the quality of the milk for baby.

Below is a list of vitamins needed for the breastfeeding mom:

**Vitamin D** – If mother and infant are not exposed to sunlight or have a diet low in vitamin D, breastfed infants need to be supplemented 5-7.5 $\mu$g/day.

**Vitamin K** – Very low risk for developing hemorrhagic disease, but all infants are given 0.5-1 mg injection of 1-2 mg oral vitamin K at birth.

**Iron** – Is usually adequate for six months, unless infant is supplemented with food too quickly. Solid food may decrease iron absorption and the diet may need to be supplemented.

**Vitamin E** – Is present in high concentrations in colostrum (8 mg/L) and decreased to three to four mg/L in mature milk. Vitamin E concentration in breast milk is responsive to maternal intake; supplementing the infant is usually not necessary, provided the mother has adequate intake.

**Vitamin C** – Usually found in adequate concentrations of about 100 mg/L of breast milk in well-nourished mothers. An intake of less than 100 mg/day may decrease milk content, but doses over 100 mg/day will not increase it. Vitamin C content in breast milk is eight to ten times higher than maternal plasma concentration.

**Vitamin K** – The quantity of vitamin K in breast milk is approximately 0.8 to 1.0 mg/L, and this can be increased to 60 mg/L with maternal supplementation of 5 mg/day. Vitamin K supplementation for newborns may be recommended for infants at risk for hemorrhagic disease. A single intramuscular (IM) dose of 1 to 5 mg IM can be given to the mother 12 to 24 hours before delivery; 0.5 to 1 mg can be given within one hour of birth, or 2 mg orally can be given to the infant. Higher doses may be needed if the mother has been taking anticoagulants.

**Thiamine** – Is present in early milk at a low concentration of 20 mg/L, but the concentration increases significantly in mature milk to 175-250 mg/L, which is adequate for the infant. Riboflavin concentrations are high in early milk and decrease to 400-600 mg/L in mature milk. The amount of niacin present is dependent upon maternal intake, rising from 0.5 mg/L in early milk, to 1.8 to 2.0 mg/L in mature milk, and possibly reaching as high as 6 mg/L with higher intake.

**Vitamin B6** – Starts low in colostrum and increases as much as ten-fold from 0.09 to 0.31 mg/L in mature milk. Vitamin B6 levels in breast milk increase with increased maternal intake, but may be reduced in women who have been using oral contraceptives for an extended period of time.

**Vitamin B12 and Folate** – These nutrients are usually found in excess because when they are secreted, they are bound to whey proteins. In well-nourished mothers, vitamin B12 concentrations are adequate (0.5 to 1.0 mg/L) and supplementation has little effect. However, levels as low as 0.05 to 0.75 mg/L have been reported in cases of women who were strict vegetarians, malnourished, or had hypothyroid-induced pernicious anemia. Infant supplementation would be recommended in such cases. Folate concentrations usually remain adequate in breast milk in spite of maternal plasma concentration or intake. The average folate concentration in breast milk ranges from 80 to 140 mg/L.

**Minerals** – Unlike vitamins, minerals do not seem to correlate with maternal intake or maternal plasma levels. Phosphorous seems to be highest in early milk, at 147 mg/L, decreasing to 107 mg/L in mature milk. Calcium increases from 259 mg/L to 290 mg/L and magnesium increases from 248 mg/L to 330 mg/L. It has been speculated that these three minerals in these concentrations are important in bone remodeling occurring in infancy.

Copper, iron, and zinc concentrations seem to be strongly related to liver stores of the mother accumulated during the third trimester. Maternal intake has very little effect on them. Copper and iron concentrations start high in early milk, leveling off to 0.3 mg/L of each. Zinc also starts higher (4 mg/L), declining to 1.1 mg/L at six months postpartum, and decreasing still to 0.5 mg/L after one year. Both iron and zinc have a high bioavailability in breast milk, but the bioavailability of copper is unknown.

Manganese declines from 6 mg/L after one month of lactation to 3 mg/L after three and six months, but is much better absorbed than the manganese found in infant formulas.

Selenium is strongly influenced by maternal selenium status. It tends to be high early in lactation (40 mg/L), decreasing in mature milk.

Iodine in breast milk varies according to maternal intake and geographic region. In iodine-sufficient areas, the breast milk content is approximately 150 mg/L, and in iodine-deficient areas it can be as low as 15 mg/L.

# Vitamin Deficiencies, Hormones and Depression

A lack of nutrients is one of the most frequent, but least recognized, causes of depression. A correlation can be drawn between nutritional deficiencies and depression. According to the *Encyclopedia of Natural Medicine*, "A deficiency of any single nutrient can alter brain function and lead to depression, anxiety, and other mental disorders." The connection between depression and vitamin and minerals deficiencies and hormone balance is often missed. The effect of nutritional deficiencies on brain chemistry cannot be understated.

Let's explore one important connection between hormone balance and nutritional deficiencies by looking at serotonin for example. Serotonin is a hormone found naturally in the human brain which helps to regulate moods, sleep, and anxiety and relieves depression and a key neurotransmitter for delivering emotional impulses to the brain. Science has linked this disease with low levels of serotonin in the brain. Many factors affect the level of serotonin in the brain such as stress levels, diet, exercise and exposure to sunlight; by increasing the levels of serotonin in the brain, science has been able to treat many types of depression and other related disorders. Increasing the levels of serotonin by eating healthier and getting the nutrition you need is a great way to help with depression symptoms.

## *B Vitamins*

One of the most common deficiencies in people with depression is a lack of one or more of the B vitamins. Research has shown a strong connection between deficiency of this vitamin and experiencing depression. The B vitamins are powerful regulators of mood. Some of the clinical effects of insufficient vitamin B complex are mood changes, insomnia and changes in appetite. As a group, the B vitamins play an important role both in alleviating depression and in relieving the anxiety and restlessness which often accompanies it.

Looking at these B vitamins individually you can get a better picture of their importance and see how they can affect depression.

**Vitamin B12** – The mental changes caused by deficiency of B12 can range from difficulty in concentrating or memory impairment, to mental and physical fatigue and low moods all the way to irritability, depression, mania and psychosis. Vitamin B12 also plays an important role in the production of certain brain chemicals such as serotonin, which is important in regulating mood and other brain function. Supplementation of folic acid and B12 often produces dramatic results in people who are depressed because of deficiencies.

**Vitamin B6 (Pyridoxine)** – Is commonly very low in people who are depressed and is associated with central nervous system problems and is the one implicated most in treatment of cause and treatment of mood disorders. This vitamin aids in the processing of amino acids, which are the building blocks of all proteins and is needed in the manufacture of serotonin, melatonin and dopamine. Deficiency can disrupt formation of neurotransmitters because this nutrient is essential for converting tryptophan to serotonin.

**Vitamin B5 (Pantothenic Acid)** – Is very important for the proper functioning of the nervous system. A deficiency can cause depression, fatigue, chronic stress and allergies. Vitamin B5 is needed for hormone formation and the uptake of amino acids and the brain chemical acetylcholine, which combine to prevent certain types of depression. Vitamin B5 is active in the formation of the neurotransmitter acetylcholine, which can be involved in some depression. The body's synthesis of acetylcholine is vital because of the neurotransmitter's role in motor behavior and memory.

**Vitamin B3 (Niacin and Niacinamide)** – Subclinical deficiencies of vitamin B3 can produce anxiety, agitation, apprehension, fatigue and irritability and other mental disturbances.

**Vitamin B2** – A deficiency can cause symptoms of depression.

**Vitamin B1 (Thiamine)** – Deficiency symptoms includes anxiety and mood disorders and can trigger depression and irritability. B1 is essential for metabolism of carbohydrates to give brain energy as well as body energy and nerve stimulation.

**Folate (Folic Acid)** – Folic acid deficiency has been found among people with depression. According to research depressive symptoms are the most common neuropsychiatric manifestation of a deficiency in folate. Folate lowers brain 5-HT (5-hydroxytryptamine: the brain hormone serotonin) and low levels of serotonin are associated with depression. Another concern is that folate deficiency may specifically affect central monoamine metabolism and aggravate depressive disorders. Folate deficiency also can limit the body's ability to convert folic acid from the diet to L-methylfolate. This is important because L-methylfolate is the only form of folate used by the brain to correct a neurotransmitter imbalance linked to depression.

## *Antioxidant Vitamins*

**Vitamin C** – Vitamin C deficiency causes chronic depression, irritability, fatigue and the "blues." A deficiency also hampers our ability to handle all types of physical and mental stress. Vitamin C is needed by the adrenal glands to synthesize hormones. Research shows that 1,000 milligrams of vitamin C taken daily helped those deal with psychological stress better than those who did not. The body tends to absorb vitamins better in natural form, so eating foods that are rich in vitamin C is your best bet.

**Vitamin E** – People with depression are shown to have lower serum vitamin E concentrations. It is important if you are depressed to consume enough vitamin E. Vitamin E also reduces free radicals in the body and boosts the immune system.

**Vitamin D3** – Enhances positive affect (mood) and is a useful treatment for SAD (Seasonal Affective Disorder). It has been suggested SAD may be due to changing levels of vitamin D3, the hormone of sunlight, leading to changes in brain serotonin.

## *Minerals*

**Magnesium** – Low magnesium levels appear to be associated with psychological changes and depressive issues. It is a critical mineral used in sending messages along your nerves. Deficiency can result in depressive symptoms along with anxiety, confusion, agitation, and hallucinations. Most diets do not include enough magnesium, and stress can actually contribute to magnesium depletion.

**Calcium** – Insufficient levels of calcium affect the central nervous system. These low levels cause nervousness, apprehension, irritability, and numbness.

**Zinc** – Inadequate levels of zinc result in apathy, lack of appetite, and lethargy. When zinc is low, copper in the body can increase to toxic levels, resulting in paranoia and fearfulness.

**Iron** – Depression is often a symptom of continuous iron deficiency. Other symptoms from low iron are exhaustion, weakness, lack of appetite and headaches.

**Manganese** – Manganese supports the B-complex vitamins and vitamin C. A deficiency may contribute to depression stemming from low levels of the neurotransmitters serotonin and norepinephrine. Manganese also helps prevent mood swings caused from blood sugar issues.

**Potassium** – Depletion is frequently associated with depression, tearfulness, weakness, and fatigue. One study found that depressed people were more likely to have decreased intracellular potassium.

## The Safety of Supplements

Vitamin C and the B-complex vitamins discussed above are all water-soluble. This means that they won't accumulate in your body or be stored for future use. Amounts above and beyond your current nutritional needs are dumped into your urine. As a result, there is no danger of overdose. Unlike water-soluble vitamins, minerals can be stored in your tissues so you want to be careful to only take the recommended dose since accumulation of minerals in the body can be dangerous. For therapeutic doses you will want to consult a healthcare provider who specializes in this or seek the advice of a qualified nutrition consultant.

**Omega-3 Fatty Acids** – Many diets are lacking enough of the necessary omega-3 oils and this has been linked to depression. Scientists believe that a lack of essential fatty acids (especially omega-3s) combined with an excess of saturated fats and animal fatty acids in diets can lead to the formation of cell membranes that are much less fluid. This loss of fluidity affects the physical properties of brain cell membranes and directly influences neurotransmitter synthesis, uptake of serotonin and other neurotransmitters, and signal transmission, enzymes that break down serotonin and other neurotransmitters such as epinephrine, dopamine and norepinephrine.

**S-adenosyl- L-methionine (SAM or SAMe)** – It is a supplement used for depression. SAMe has been studied for decades internationally and is approved as a prescription drug in Spain, Italy, Russia and Germany. Europeans have used it, primarily for depression and arthritis. Normally, the brain manufactures all the SAMe it needs from the amino acid methionine but SAM synthesis is impaired in depressed patients. Our diet yields insufficient quantities of SAMe and our bodies can only generate a small amount of SAMe. Therefore, SAMe levels are to be increased through dietary supplementation, if that is necessary. A number of clinical studies suggest that SAMe is one of the most effective natural antidepressants.

**Tryptophan** – As we discussed before, serotonin is a very important brain biochemical and must be present at optimal levels to prevent depression. Tryptophan supplementation has been shown to increase the levels of serotonin and melatonin in the brain. Many depressed individuals have been found to have low tryptophan and serotonin levels. European studies have shown that L-tryptophan is of value in relieving depression. Unfortunately, other studies have given mixed results as to the effectiveness of tryptophan in depression. Tryptophan works much more effectively if used with vitamin B6 and the niacinamide form of vitamin B3 to help block the kynurenine pathway to provide better results.

Tryptophan can found in certain foods sources as well, such as milk, turkey, chicken, fish, cooked dried beans and peas, brewer's yeast, peanut butter, nuts, and soybeans. Eat plenty of these foods together with carbohydrates such as potatoes, pasta, rice and this will help the brain's uptake of tryptophan. Foods such as bananas, walnuts and pineapples are a good source of serotonin. To convert tryptophan to serotonin, the body must have adequate levels of folic acid, vitamin B-6, magnesium, niacin, and glutamine.

**5-Hydroxytryptophan (5-HTP)** – The use of 5-HTP is felt by some to be more effective than the use of tryptophan for depression because it is one step closer to serotonin lineage than tryptophan. It is preferred for the treatment of depression over tryptophan by some. 5-HTP is extracted from the seed of an African plant (Griffonia simplicifolia) and not synthesized with bacteria so there isn't the concern for contamination. Also only three percent of an oral dose of tryptophan is converted to serotonin, over seventy percent of an oral dose of 5-HTP is converted to serotonin. 5-HTP causes an increase in levels of endorphin and other neurotransmitters that are often decreased in cases of depression. 5-HTP also increases serotonin levels. Thus, it is much more effective for depression.

Dietary modification and vitamin and mineral supplementation in some cases reduce the severity of depression and can result in an overall improvement in well-being. The nutritional treatment of depression includes dietary modifications, supportive treatment with vitamins and minerals, and supplementation with specific amino acids, which are precursors to neurotransmitters. Correcting deficiencies, when present, often relieves depression. However, even if a deficiency cannot be demonstrated, nutritional supplementation can still improve symptoms and overall wellness.

# ACSS Food Suggestions and Serving Sizes

After giving birth, it is a great time to re-evaluate your nutritional needs. An adequate diet is especially important to help ensure your health and to supply you with the energy necessary to care for your new baby. Remember to drink plenty of liquids. Drink to satisfy your thirst, but be sure to drink eight to ten glasses of liquid every day. Below are guides to food groups and serving sizes for postpartum mothers.

To help you navigate your nutritional needs and combat fatigue, depression, below are the ACSS Tried and True Food Suggestions and Serving Sizes.

## *Protein-Rich Foods*

Below are the recommended minimum daily servings of lean sources of protein:

Choose *seven* if you are breastfeeding; and *five* if you are bottle feeding.

One Serving Equals:
- 1 oz. fish or other seafood
- 1 oz. beef, chicken, turkey or pork
- 1 cooked egg
- 1/2 cup cooked dry beans (pinto, soy, lentils, kidney)
- 3 oz. tofu
- 1/4 cup peanuts, 2 Tbsp. peanut butter, 1/3 cup other nuts
- 1/4 cup sunflower seeds

## *Milk Products*

Below are the recommended minimum daily servings of calcium-rich milk products:

Choose *three* if you are breastfeeding; and *three* if you are bottle feeding.

One Serving Equals:
- 8 oz. fluid milk or yogurt
- 1-1/2 oz. hard cheeses (jack, cheddar, mozzarella, Swiss)
- 1-1/2 cups ice cream or frozen yogurt
- 1/2 cup ricotta cheese

- 4 Tbsp. Parmesan cheese
- 1 cup pudding or custard (made of milk)
- 2 cups cottage cheese

# Breads, Cereals and Grains

Below are the recommended minimum daily servings of breads, cereals and grains:

Choose *seven* if you are breastfeeding; and *six-seven* if you are bottle feeding.

One serving equals:
- 1 slice bread or dinner roll
- 1/2 English muffin, 1/2 bagel
- 1/2 small pita or 1/2 hamburger bun
- 1/2 cup pasta, noodles, or rice
- 1/2 cup cooked cereal
- 1 muffin, whole wheat
- 1 small tortilla, corn or wheat
- 3/4 cup cold cereal, bran flakes, Cheerios
- 6 saltine-type crackers or 12 wheat crackers
- 3 cups popcorn
- 1/2 cup granola
- 1 small pancake or waffle
- 2 breadsticks (4"x 1/2")

# Vitamin C-Rich Fruits and Vegetables

Below are the recommended minimum daily servings of vitamin C-rich fruits and vegetables:

Choose *one* if you are breastfeeding; and *one* if you are bottle feeding.

One serving equals:
- 6 oz. orange, tomato, grapefruit juice or vegetable juice cocktail
- 1 fresh orange, kiwi, mango, guava or lemon, 2 tangerines, 1/2 cup papaya
- 1/2 cup strawberries or cantaloupe
- 1/2 cup broccoli, Brussels sprouts, cauliflower, snow peas or bell peppers

- 2 medium tomatoes, 1/2 cup tomato puree or 1/2 cup cooked cabbage
- 1/2 medium grapefruit
- 2 Tbsp. hot chili peppers

## Vitamin A-Rich Fruits and Vegetables

Below are the recommended minimum daily servings of vitamin A-rich fruits and vegetables:

Choose *one* if you are breastfeeding; and *one* if you are bottle feeding

One serving equals:
- 1 small carrot
- 6 oz. apricot nectar or vegetable juice
- 3 fresh apricots
- 1/2 cup cooked greens (mustard, kale, spinach, bok choy, chard, collards)
- 1/4 mango or cantaloupe
- 1/2 cup sweet potatoes, pumpkin, yams, winter squash, 2 medium tomatoes
- 1 cup fresh spinach or parsley
- 2 Tbsp. hot chili peppers

## Other Fruits and Vegetables

Below are the recommended minimum daily servings of other fruits and vegetables:

Choose *three* if you are breastfeeding; and *three* if you are bottle feeding.

One serving equals:
- 6 oz. fruit juice
- 1/2 cup sliced: apple, banana, berries, cucumber, grapes, peaches, pears, corn, peas, potatoes, pineapple, green beans, zucchini, watermelon, mushrooms, cherries, onions
- 2 medium plums, 1/2 cup applesauce
- 1 medium nectarine
- 1/4 cup raisins
- 1 cup lettuce

## *Unsaturated Fats*

Below are the recommended minimum daily servings of unsaturated fats:

Choose *three* if you are breastfeeding; and *three* if you are bottle feeding.

One serving equals:
- 1 tsp. margarine, mayonnaise, or vegetable oil (canola, safflower, corn, olive)
- 1 tsp. salad dressing (mayonnaise-based)
- 1 Tbsp. salad dressing (oil-based)
- 1/8 avocado
- 10 small or 5 large olives

## *Saturated Fat*

Below are the recommended minimum daily servings of unsaturated fats:

*Use sparingly!*

One serving equals:
- 1 Tbsp. butter
- 1 slice bacon
- 2 Tbsp. sour cream
- 1 Tbsp. cream cheese

# Breastfeeding

Breast milk is best for your baby, and the benefits of breastfeeding extend well beyond your baby's basic nutrition. In addition to containing all the vitamins and nutrients your baby needs in the first six months of life, breast milk is packed with disease-fighting substances that protect your baby from illness. That's one reason the American Academy of Pediatrics recommends exclusive breastfeeding for the first six months of your baby's life, although any amount of breastfeeding is beneficial for your baby, be it six weeks or six months!

Breastfeeding's protection against illness lasts well beyond your baby's breastfeeding stage, as well. Studies have shown that breastfeeding can reduce a child's risk of developing certain childhood cancers. Scientists believe the antibodies in breast milk may give a baby's immune system a boost. Breastfeeding may also help children avoid diseases that occur later in life, such as diabetes (type 1 and type 2), high cholesterol, and inflammatory bowel disease. In fact, preemies given breast milk as babies are less likely to have high blood pressure by the time they're teenagers.

The first two hours after birth is the perfect time to initiate breastfeeding. It is known as the "quiet alert state." After the fatigue from birth, adjustment to lights, temperature change and new sounds, your baby will be alert, looking around, chewing on his/her fists and naturally rooting and looking for the comfort of your breast. Now is the time for your little one's first time to nurse!

It is best to have the baby unbundled and skin-to-skin if possible, snuggled within your arm and against your body. This opportunity also gives you, the first time mom, confidence in your ability to breastfeed your baby. It stimulates the hormones that cause your uterus to clamp down and contract and remain firm after your birth. These contractions, called "afterpains" will occur the first few days after birth when you breastfeed your baby. Mothers who have had other children will have afterpains that are especially more uncomfortable because their uterus needs to work harder to contract and to return to its non-pregnant state.

As mentioned earlier, the first milk present at birth is called colostrum. Colostrum is critical in boosting your baby's immune system and in encouraging the passage of the first stool. Colostrum, although present only in small amounts, provides concentrated and sufficient nutrition for your baby.

Supplements are not necessary.

Lactation is based on supply and demand. The more milk your baby removes from your breast, the more milk will be made. The suckling action of your baby at your breast causes levels of your hormones to increase, thus initiating the let-down reflex. Your baby should be nursing 8-12 times in a 24-hour period. Until your milk comes in, your baby needs frequent feedings of your colostrum. When your milk comes in by the third postpartum day, a good feeding every few hours will help ensure an abundant milk supply.

Before putting your baby to breast, be sure you are in a comfortable position, pillows everywhere for support, prior to putting your baby to breast. Proper positioning is everything to help alleviate sore nipples and improper latch on. Discomfort while breastfeeding is usually due to improper latching or positioning at the breast. Frequent nursing does not cause sore nipples.

The trick to breastfeeding is getting the baby to latch on well. A baby who latches on well, gets milk well. A baby who latches on poorly has difficulty getting milk.

*What is a good latch?*
- Wide open mouth (nearly a 180 degree opening at the corner of your baby's mouth).
- Lips turned out, not rolled in.
- Baby's chin touches the breast.
- Baby's tongue should be under the nipple.

*Signals to remove your baby from the breast and re-try the latch:*
- You are experiencing strong discomfort or pain.
- Baby sucks in his cheek pads with each suckle.
- Baby makes clicking or smacking noises.
- Baby does not suck and swallow rhythmically.

After the first 24 hours of birth, babies tend to be very sleepy. If your baby has not been to breast after a three-hour period (from the beginning of the last feeding) unswaddle, talk to the baby, rub his or her back. At this point, your baby should become interested in taking your breast to feed. Encourage your baby to have a good feeding each time he/she nurses. When your baby has released the nipple, or when he/she stops swallowing, burp him/her. After burping your baby may regain interest and take the second breast. If babe only nurses for a short time, be sure to start on that side at the next feeding.

Scheduled or timed feedings are discouraged. Be aware of your baby's hunger cues. Be aware of feeding readiness cues, especially if your baby is sleepy; e.g., rapid eye movements under eyelids, sucking movements of the mouth and tongue, hand-to-mouth movements, body movements, small sounds, etc. Crying is a late sign of hunger.

Frequent feedings are encouraged during your baby's early newborn period to build milk supply, feeding at least 8-12 times in 24 hours. Be re-assured that frequent nursing does not cause sore nipples. Sore nipples are due to improper positioning and latch onto the breast. Encourage baby-led feedings. Encourage nursing on one side until baby finishes, offering the second breast and feeding according to your baby's interest. Discourage time limits at the breast. Your baby will typically come off the breast independently, fall asleep or appear disinterested in nursing when he has finished feeding at a breast. Method to end a feeding (if necessary) is by breaking suction between your baby's mouth and nipple. Do not let baby pull off nipple.

*Signs of adequate milk supply*
- Mouth movements, drawing in of areola, and audible swallow
- Adequate weight gain of four to six oz./week
- Six wet/heavy diapers every 24 hours AFTER DAY FOUR
- Four or more bowel movements every 24 hours AFTER DAY FOUR

The first days of your milk production are critical for determining whether you will have an adequate milk supply for your baby. If little milk is removed from your breast, the resulting pressure causes your breast to slow down its milk production. If no milk is removed, your mild production will stop entirely. To make sure you have a generous milk supply depends on a vigorous nursing baby or an effective breast pump that drains at least one breast every few hours around the clock.

If you find the breastfeeding process difficult or your baby is having difficulty latching, it can be an emotionally and psychologically taxing experience. To help manage a smooth transition, consider reaching out to a lactation consultant, they can make scheduled appointments at your home to help guide you.

## Engorgement

At two to three days postpartum, your breasts will become engorged or swollen. Believe it or not, this IS a positive sign: it is caused by the increased flow of blood to the breasts and the start of your milk production. You're producing milk to feed your baby, and soon, with your baby's help, you'll produce the right amount. For some moms, their breasts only become slightly full, for others they feel very swollen, tender, throbbing and even lumpy. Sometimes the swelling may extend into your armpit. Engorgement can cause your nipples to flatten, making it difficult for your baby to latch on to nurse. The problem usually lessens within 24 to 48 hours, but the swelling and discomfort may worsen if nursing is too brief or infrequent or if your baby's suck is ineffective. If engorgement is unrelieved by nursing or pumping, milk production declines and will eventually stop altogether.

The degree of engorgement usually lessens with each child. First-time moms often suffer more from engorgement than women who are nursing their second or third child, because the time it takes for the mature milk to "come in" seems to shorten with each child.

*Treatment Measures for Engorgement*

- Wear a supportive nursing bra, even during the night while you sleep. Be sure your bra fits properly and is not too tight. Avoid under-wire bras, do not bind your breasts - this can lead to plugged or blocked ducts.
- Nurse frequently. Try to nurse at least 8-12 times in 24 hours - every 1 ½ - 2 hours during the day, with no more than a 3 hour stretch at night.
- Try to nurse for at least 15 minutes on the first side before offering the second. Do not set time limits on time spent at the breast.
- Nurse baby with only a diaper on (skin- to -skin contact will stimulate sucking).
- Vary nursing positions to help promote drainage of the breast.
- Wear breast shells (with holes for air circulation) for 20 minutes between feedings.
- Lie flat on your back between feedings so that your breasts are elevated.

Apply cold compresses to your breasts and under your arms between feedings. Cold can help reduce swelling. Use a layer of fabric between the compress and the skin. Bags of frozen vegetables or a disposable diaper that you dampen and put in the freezer for 20 minutes work just as well as the ice packs that you purchase at the drugstore. Apply cold compresses for 15-20 minutes off and on for one to two hours.

The use of heat immediately before nursing can help the milk let-down. Taking a warm shower, leaning over a basin of warm water, soaking in a warm bath, or applying warm compresses or a heating pad may help. Moist heat is best. Gentle breast massage can also help the milk flow more readily.

If the nipple and areola are swollen, don't try to nurse without softening them up first. Hand express or pump a little milk from your breast to soften the nipple and areola before trying to nurse. Gently massage the breast before nursing. If you use an electric pump, set it on MINIMUM and gradually increase the pressure after the milk begins to flow. You may not be able to turn it up to maximum, but try to increase the pressure as much as you comfortably can. Most pumps work better on the higher settings, but if the breast and nipple tissue is extremely tender, don't try to increase the suction. Apply a few drops of olive oil to your nipple and areola before pumping to help prevent friction while pumping.

Be careful about the type of pump you use. Many of the small inexpensive electric pumps, can damage your tissue, since engorged breasts bruise easily due to the increased blood volume. If you don't have access to a high quality pump which cycles automatically, you may want to stick with manual expression. Even with manual expression or massage, be very, very gentle.

If your breasts remain full, knotty, and tender after nursing, you may want to pump for 5-10 minutes to remove all the milk that comes out quickly and easily. Don't be afraid that nursing or pumping will increase your milk supply and make the engorgement worse. At this early stage, when your milk is just coming in, remember that the fullness is a buildup of other fluids (blood and lymph) as well as milk. Removing the milk will relieve the pressure and reduce the swelling, softening the areola and making it easier for the baby to latch on.

You may want to use cabbage leaf compresses if the above suggestions don't bring you enough relief. This sounds really strange, but this is a remedy that has been used for over a hundred years with much success. No one is exactly sure why it works, but since it is inexpensive, safe, and effective, you may want to give it a try.

*Here's what to do:*
1. Buy plain green cabbage.
1. Rinse and dry leaves. Put them in the refrigerator.
2. Remove base of hard core vein and gently pound leaves.
3. Wrap around breast and areola, leaving nipple exposed. The leaves fit nicely around the breast, and the cold feels good.
4. Cover entire breast, and if needed, the area under your arms.
5. Change every 30 minutes or sooner if they become wilted.
6. Check your breasts often and as soon as you feel the milk beginning to drip, or if your breasts feel 'different', remove leaves and try to nurse or pump.
7. Re-apply as needed (up to three times between feedings). Check OFTEN as over use can cause a decrease in your milk supply.

If pain and swelling persist, ask your healthcare provider about use of an anti-inflammatory drug compatible with breastfeeding. Often Advil (two tablets taken three or four times a day, every six to eight hours with food) will be helpful. Tylenol (acetaminophen) may also be used for pain relief.

Sage tea (available at health food stores) is a powerful herb that contains a natural form of estrogen and may decrease your milk supply. Drinking a cup at bedtime for a night or two may help in cases of severe engorgement. As with cabbage leaves, monitor breast changes often as over use can decrease your supply.

Call your healthcare provider if your temperature rises over 101 F, or if you develop localized pain or flu-like symptoms. Even if you develop a breast infection, breastfeeding can and should continue.

Remember that engorgement usually subsides within 24-48 hours, so hang in there. Severe engorgement that is not treated promptly may take up to a week to resolve, and there is a greater risk of developing an infection. During this uncomfortable period, take comfort in the fact that most mothers who experience engorgement usually have more than adequate milk supplies once the initial period of discomfort is over. Lactation Consultants worry much more about mothers who don't experience some degree of breast fullness during the postpartum period than those who do.

It is also important to note that the uncomfortable fullness you experience in the first few days after your baby's birth is due to a hormonal rush that will never again be duplicated. You may experience a degree of engorgement later on if your baby sleeps a long stretch for the first time, or if you are separated from your infant, but you will never again have the same hormonal response that you will have immediately after his birth.

*Resources for breastfeeding:*
- La Leche League International (www.llli.org)
- *The Breastfeeding Book: Everything You Need to Know About Nursing Your Child from Birth Through Weaning* by Martha Sears and William Sears
- *The Womanly Art of Breastfeeding* (La Leche League International Book) by Diane Wiessinger
- *The Complete Book of Breastfeeding*, 4th edition: The Classic Guide by Sally Wendkos Olds and Laura Marks M.D.
- *Ina May's Guide to Breastfeeding* by Ina May Gaskin

# *Mastitis*

Mastitis occurs when bacteria enter your breast through a break or crack in the skin of your nipple or through the opening to the milk ducts in your nipple. Bacteria from your skin's surface and baby's mouth enter the milk duct and can multiply — leading to pain, redness and swelling of the breast as infection progresses.

Mastitis is often caused by Staphylococcus aureus and Escherichia coli bacteria. It is an unwelcome guest, especially to first time moms who have a difficult enough time trying to establish a breastfeeding routine with their baby. It is also unwelcome to those of you who have already experienced cracked nipples, have thin or sensitive skin, engorgement or a weakened immune system. Mastitis is often preceded by engorgement, plugged milk ducts or cracked and bleeding nipples.

Mastitis needs to be differentiated from a plugged or blocked duct, because the plugged or blocked duct does not need treatment with antibiotics, whereas mastitis often, but not always, does require treatment with antibiotics. A blocked or plugged duct presents as a painful, swollen, firm mass in the breast. The skin overlying the blocked duct is often red, similar to what happens during mastitis, but less intense. Mastitis is usually associated with fever and more intense pain as well. However, it is not always easy to distinguish between a mild mastitis and a severe blocked duct. A blocked duct, can progress to mastitis.

*Symptoms of mastitis include:*
- A red, sore spot or "hot spot" on your breast
- Breast tenderness or warmth to the touch
- Swelling of the breast
- General malaise or feeling ill
- Overall, flu-like symptoms
- Fever of 101F or 38.3 C or greater
- Red lines following the troubled milk duct's path

Because many healthcare providers will prescribe antibiotics, it is up to the mother to find, in addition to the antibiotics, other remedies and comfort measures to help shorten the episode of mastitis, ease the pain and help to continue to breastfeed your baby.

There are a number of self-care remedies for mastitis. Resting, continuing breastfeeding and drinking extra fluids can help your body overcome the breast infection. If you are prescribed an antibiotic, the course of therapy will usually be ten to fourteen days of antibiotics. Even though you may feel better after 48 to 72 hours of taking the antibiotics, be sure to finish the antibiotic regimen to ensure your breast infection is resolved.

*To relieve your pain and discomfort:*

- Be sure to maintain your breastfeeding routine. Yes, you can still breastfeed your baby with a breast infection. It is safe for you and for your baby. It is also recommended by the La Leche League to continue breastfeeding on the affected breast through mastitis to help shorten the episode of the infection and avoid abscesses. Mastitis need never be the reason to discontinue breastfeeding your baby.
- Avoid prolonged engorgement before breastfeeding your baby. You need to reduce the fullness as much as possible at each feeding to ease the inflammation and expel any milk plugs that may be present. Some babies may be reluctant to breastfeed on the infected breast because of elevated sodium content in the milk. If your baby cannot be persuaded to nurse, you need to express milk to keep your breast soft.
- Use different positions to breastfeed your baby; sometimes the same position causes pressure points on a certain area of the breast, thus causing a plugged duct which can lead to mastitis. Be sure you are in a good and comfortable position before your baby latches on!
- Drink plenty of fluids! Did I mention this before? This is important enough to repeat!
- If it is too painful to breastfeed on the affected breast and/or your breast is too sore to have babe latch on, you can pump and hand express your milk.
- If you have difficulty emptying a portion of your breast, apply warm compresses to your breasts, take a warm shower, or kneel in your tub filled with warm water and submerge your breasts before breastfeeding your baby or pumping
- Wear a good supportive bra.
- While waiting for the antibiotics to take effect, take a mild pain reliever such as acetaminophen (Tylenol, others) or ibuprofen (Motrin, Advil, others).

You can reduce your chances of getting mastitis by fully draining the milk from your breast while breastfeeding. Allow your baby to completely empty one breast before switching to the other breast during feeding. If your baby nurses only a few minutes on the second breast, or not at all, start breastfeeding on that breast at your next feeding.

Alternate the breast you offer first at each feeding, and change the position you use to breastfeed from one feeding to the next. Make sure your babe latches on properly before each feeding. If your baby is not latched on properly, break the suction with your finger. If baby fusses a few seconds, that is okay. This is better than you developing cracked nipples that can lead to mastitis.

Finally, do not let your baby use you as a pacifier. Babies enjoy sucking and often find comfort in suckling at the breast even when they are not hungry.

Breastfeeding your baby is one of the most fulfilling actions in the mother-infant bonding process. It should be pain free and fulfilling.

# Exercise (Mom & Baby)

Having a baby means lots of new things: lack of sleep, learning how to care for a new baby and of course dealing with the pregnancy weight you gained during pregnancy. Whether it is the furthest thing from your mind or a constant reminder every time you walk by the mirror, this section will answer your most pressing questions: When should I start exercising again? How much and for how long? When do I find the time? Can I work my abs? What is the best type of exercise for me?

And the most pressing question: How long will it take for me to lose the weight?

First and foremost remember it took nine months for your body to change and adapt, to grow life from within. Give yourself *at least* nine months to lose the weight; if not, you risk putting yourself at risk, and possibly your baby, depending on how compelled you feel to lose the weight.

## When Should I Start Exercising Again?

Most healthcare providers will give you the go-ahead after six to eight weeks to return to normal exercise. For women who gave vaginal birth, the time recommendation is usually six weeks after birth, while those who had a c-section can usually resume exercise after eight weeks. Considering that nothing is really normal after childbirth, there are exercises in the first weeks that can and will help your return to "normal" exercises that much easier.

## Light Exercises

These exercises are centered on breathing, stretching and isometric contractions.

**Kegel exercises:** Kegel exercises involve making small contractions of the muscles at the vaginal wall. These exercises can help strengthen weak pelvic muscles, which can cause bladder control issues, which are common in women postpartum.

**Walking:** With your provider's approval, short, slow walks can help prepare your body for more vigorous exercise, as well as get you fresh air. A week or two after birth, taking a series of short walks is healthy and will feel refreshing. It's best to wait until bleeding has stopped before taking really long walks or doing heavy lifting. If you feel like getting out of the house, head to a park for a short walk and then sit for a while. If we overexert ourselves by doing too much physical activity, postpartum bleeding increases. This is a message from your body asking you to slow down. If this happens, make a point of resting more over the next few days.

**Yoga**: Gentle yoga poses can be a great way to get your blood flowing while reducing stress. You may need to avoid some poses (like inversions), but basic moves like supported bridge, warrior I and pelvic tilts, are a great place to start. You may also be able to find a postpartum yoga class at a local gym or health club.

Always avoid or refrain from exercising if you experience any negative side effects. These side effects include: increased bleeding, increased low back pain, light headedness/dizziness, pain at incision (cesarean or episiotomy).

## Preparing for Abdominal Exercises

The abdominal muscles for many moms after birth, and up to the first two months, are still stretched out. Simple exercises (shown on the next page) will help new moms begin to bring their abdominals in tight against the organs. And yes, your stomach can go back to pre-baby form, but it will take the right type of exercise and more importantly the right type of nutrition to get you there (see the nutrition information for 0-2 months starting on page 177).

First, here's an overview of the muscles we're focusing on and visualizing when we do abdominal exercises.

*Anatomy of the Abdominals:*

- The **transverse abdominis** muscle is the deepest support layer and wraps horizontally around the mid-section. It is the transverse muscle that stretches the most during pregnancy and thus the first abdominal muscle to target postpartum.
- The **rectus abdominis** or "six pack muscle" is the muscle that most people associate as the "abs." This muscle runs vertically from the pelvis to the ribs and is divided into two halves. The primary function of this muscle is to bend the spine forward. These two halves sometimes split during pregnancy, to make room for the growing uterus, which is called diastasis recti.
- The **obliques** or "love handles" are scientifically known as the internal and external obliques. These muscles are used to rotate and laterally flex the spine and are the last muscles to target in a postnatal abdominal routine.

## *Postnatal Abdominal Workout (2-4 weeks postpartum):*

---

### Use Caution

Before beginning or performing any exercise, consult with your provider if you experience any pain or discomfort. This is especially important for mom's who feel pain near the cesarean incision. Always be sure to exercise within a pain free range of motion that feels right to you.

---

**All Fours Breathing** – On all fours, lift from the belly button to draw the abdominals in with an exhale and release on an inhale. This exercise will begin to strengthen the transverse abdominals. Try this 10-15 times, 3 times per day.

**Elevator Holds** – Seated in a chair, this exercise is similar to the all fours breathing. With shoulders back and down, draw the abdominals in on your exhale and then hold your muscles in while continuing to breathe. Hold this position for 30 seconds and then release. Try this two to three times per week; add in a Kegels hold to further intensify the exercise.

**Dead Bug** – Lying on your back, rotate your hips (similar to a hip thrust dance move) to slightly press lower back into the floor. Engage the abdominals to hold in this position (pull transverse in like in All Fours Breathing). Hold your arms out directly in front of and away from your chest. Inhale and lift your arms over your head and keep your abs in the same position. As you exhale, bring your arms back to chest and maintain abdominals contracted and with lower back slightly pressed to the floor. This exercise is essential to moving on to more difficult exercises. Work your way up to three sets of 15-20 reps.

## What is Diastasis Recti?

For some women, pregnancy can cause abdominal separation (also called diastasis recti), a condition where the Rectus Abdominis, or the "six-pack" muscle, spreads apart at the body's midline, the linea alba. Separation occurs because as the uterus puts pressure on the abdominals, and combined with pregnancy hormones that soften the abdominal wall, you may have separation. This separation can occur at any time during the last half of the pregnancy.

Abdominal separation reduces the integrity and functional strength of the abdominal wall and can aggravate lower back pain and pelvic instability. Separation in a previous pregnancy significantly increases the probability, and severity, of the condition in subsequent pregnancies. Women expecting more than one baby, very petite women, those with a pronounced sway back, or with poor abdominal muscle tone are at increased risk. Genetics also plays a big role.

Unfortunately, flurries of misconception swirl around the issue of abdominal reconditioning—and particularly abdominal separation/diastasis recti—after pregnancy. You're likely to encounter a broad range of contradictory opinions and advice about how to recondition your abdominal wall and how to restore the midline after childbirth. Some of these assertions can cause unnecessary alarm, while another common piece of advice—do a lot of "crunches"—can actually worsen abdominal separation.

*What are some common Myths about Postpartum Abdominal Conditioning?*

- Abdominal separation/diastasis recti causes permanent damage to your midline.
- Abdominal muscles will never flatten after separation/diastasis.
- Abdominal separation/diastasis recti requires surgical repair.
- The abdominal muscles will always be weaker after childbirth.
- Everyone should wait for at least six weeks after delivery before beginning a postnatal reconditioning program.

*None of these statements are true!*

Keep in mind that women who hold themselves up as living examples of the inevitable and lasting damage pregnancy has done to their bodies may not have had the benefits of a systematic postpartum exercise program designed by an expert in reconditioning after pregnancy.

---

**Abdominal Separation/Diastasis Recti Test**

This simple self-test will help you determine if you have abdominal separation and how severe it is.

1. Lie on your back with your knees bent, and the soles of your feet on the floor.
2. Place one hand behind your head and the other hand on your abdomen, with your fingertips across your midline—parallel with your waistline— at the level of your belly button.
3. With your abdominal wall relaxed, gently press your fingertips into your abdomen.
4. Roll your upper body off the floor into a "crunch," making sure that your ribcage moves closer to your pelvis.
5. Move your fingertips back and forth across your midline, feeling for the right and left sides of your Rectus Abdominis muscle.

If you feel a gap between the abdominals, or a space where you can insert your fingers and feel as if you can keep pushing down than you have diastasis recti.

---

Not to worry, many women have this, and it can be made better, and not worse, even during pregnancy.  Make sure you mention it to your healthcare provider at your next visit and also refer to the pregnancy abdominal workout at www.9monthsin9monthsout.com for how to keep your abdominals strong for all nine months! Many of these exercises can even prevent or help reverse the separation.

# Stress Management

Your friends and family members weren't kidding when they told you how tired you'd be. It does pass, especially if you've enlisted the help of your spouse or partner and those close to you. You'll learn to get the laundry done, or find a new routine with it. The dishes may pile up, but you'll figure out how to get to them.

You'll start building a routine. If you'd like assistance building one, please visit our website at www.9monthsin9monthsout.com for helpful tips and mom-tested tricks of time management.

*A few tips to help ease the transition of becoming Mom:*

**Create a relaxation ritual for yourself** - Just as you did during pregnancy, take a bath, put on some soothing music, even take a few moments to have a hot cup of tea by yourself.

**Allow others to help** - Let them bring lunches and dinners over, don't be shy about laundry (there is a lot of it).

**Learn to let things go** – Stress is mostly what we make of it.

**Breathe** – Remember the reverse pattern breathing from earlier? Take three long, slow, deep breaths in and up, out and down. Give yourself time.

**Get moving** – As soon as you can get out for a walk with your baby. Get moving and let the endorphins back into your body. You may be tired, but even a few minutes a day will naturally lower your stress.

**Aromatherapy** – Light a lavender scented candle; it's naturally soothing for you and your baby.

Enjoy the process of becoming Mom. It's a beautiful experience!

# Parental Skills

If you have no experience in caring for a baby, consider taking a childcare class offered in your local community. Your county government website should have links set up for Community Services and Classes. Ask your healthcare provider or other mothers.

Your local Department of Social Services can help lead you to some wonderful child care providers should you need to start thinking about going back to work. Each state carries different requirements for licensed and un-licensed providers. Do your research, ask around – ask every parent you see with small children as they will give you the best answers on how they've felt about certain providers.

Your local hospital will also have classes on breastfeeding and parenting programs. Classes will range in content and price, but take the time to investigate the right class for you to help build your knowledge and skills as a parent.

## *Shaken Baby Syndrome*

One of the biggest concerns during your baby's early months can be Shaken Baby Syndrome. We're tired. We're stressed. We just want the baby to stop crying because we don't understand yet. Always handle your baby with care!

Never shake an infant or small child. Shaken Baby Syndrome, also known as Abusive Head Trauma, is a serious condition that can be fatal or leave devastating permanent injuries. Even a few seconds of violent shaking can cause great harm to your little one.

*So, how do you soothe yourself and your baby?*
- Check to make sure your baby is not wet, hungry or running a fever.
- While sitting, hold your baby gently over your knees or against your chest and lightly pat your baby's back to see if he/she needs to burp.
- Go for a walk together.
- Try a pacifier. Sometimes the act of sucking helps soothe the child (and don't worry, pacifier habits are easy enough to break).
- Set up the swing and see if the rocking motion will help.
- Turn on some soothing music, something with less than 60 beats a minute. (Check the website www.9monthsin9monthsout.com for some free downloads.)

- Put your baby down in his or her crib and walk away for a while; take a few deep breaths and call a friend or your mother.

Create a plan so you know what you're going to do and who to call when you feel like you've reached your limit. If you have your resources listed out in advance, you're less likely to need them!

## Love & Logic®

A great parenting/communication program to consider looking into is Love & Logic® (www.loveandlogic.com). Parents love the ease with which they can introduce the communication techniques to their households.

*Love and Logic® provides simple and practical techniques to help parents with kids of all ages:*
- Raise responsible kids
- Have more fun in their role
- Easily change their children's behavior

For example, how many times have you seen, or been a part of, the shoe battle? Little man doesn't want to put his shoes on and you need to get out the door. Usually the conversation goes something like this:
"Time to go, let's get your shoes on," says Mom.
"No."
"Yes."

And then, the battle ensues.

Using the Love & Logic method, the conversation flows like this:
"Brandon, are you going to wear your tennis shoes or your sandals today?"
"Tennis shoes."

And that's it. No battle, no fuss, no high blood pressure. Everyone is happy!

# Conclusion

Being a parent is fulfilling and challenging. It takes a family to raise a child. Setting yourself up to succeed makes the whole process more enjoyable and then, you do get to enjoy the overwhelming love while watching your child sleep.

# Month 3 & Beyond

Motherhood is the most rewarding but challenging job you will ever have. As a mom you will experience a deeper love than you have ever thought possible. You may also experience a level of mental and physical exhaustion that you have probably never experienced. At times you will wonder why you decided to become a parent and at other times you will wonder why you didn't do this sooner. You are in the middle of life altering changes and adjustments right now, and your life is changed forever. What can you do to enjoy every moment? Learn to focus on the positive and make it a daily habit.

## Postnatal Nutrition – Why Dieting is Not the Answer

Everywhere you look there is a new diet - low carb, low fat, Mediterranean, Atkins! How is anyone suppose to know what to eat, or what supplements to take? We all know that losing weight is difficult, but it doesn't have to be so hard! And once you have hit that three month mark you are probably feeling like the baby weight should be all gone…right? WRONG! As moms we know all too well how difficult losing baby weight can be, and for some of us, twenty years later we still have ten pounds of baby weight to lose!

Here we explore ways to help us lose those 10, 20 or even 30 left over pounds!

### *Know Your Body's Math*

Too many moms think the way to lose weight is to simply cut out calories. When you go on a super low calorie diet your body literally shuts down and preserves energy or fat, on the body. In order to break this cycle, you need to be consuming enough calories to give your body energy, but just shy of how many calories you are burning. When total calories equal less than calories burned, you lose weight. Not sure of what this number is, check out the internet or local nutrition store and find out what your BMR or Basal Metabolic Rate is. This number is the measure of how many calories you burn at rest. If you are exercising, or chasing after a toddler your total calorie expenditure will need to be higher than this.

Here is an example for a 140 pound mom:

Take 140 x 10 = 1400. Now add 140 to that. That gives us a total of 1,540 calories. So a woman who has recently given birth and now weights 140 pounds should consume at least 1540 calories per day, in order to lose weight. For more information about losing weight or calculating your caloric needs, check out our tools at www.9monthsin9monthsout.com.

## *Eat Every Three to Four Hours, Hungry or Not!*

Why is it that everyone thinks in order to lose weight they need to eat less? The opposite is actually true; in order to lose weight you need to eat small meals every three to four hours in order to speed up the metabolism. Skipping meals leads to food cravings, binge eating and weight gain. Why? You are more likely to overeat when you have not eaten in eight hours than when you eat something small every three to four hours. When you choose to eat less or skip a meal your body goes into "starvation mode," and your metabolism slows down to preserve energy. You gain weight because your body stores all the food you consume because it assumes you will starve yourself again. The only way to break this cycle is to eat small meals, starting with breakfast and following with mini meals every three to four hours.

## *Always Eat Protein with Your Carbohydrates!*

Carbohydrates break down into sugar, or more specifically blood sugar, which provides energy for our body. The glycemic index refers to how fast a carbohydrate will enter our blood stream and how fast it will leave our system. Simple carbs are fast-acting carbs that provide an immediate rush of energy that quickly fades. Complex carbs are longer acting carbs that take longer to digest and provide longer-lasting amounts of energy. Good sources of complex carbs are oatmeal, brown rice, whole grain pastas and sweet potatoes. However, the key here is that if you are not using the carbohydrates they will be stored as fat!

Adding protein to the mix, slows down the digestion process, aids in building muscle and losing weight, and decreases how fast the carbohydrates go into and out of your system.

## Multi-Vitamins and Why We All Need Them

It would be ideal if moms got all the nutrients needed from our food, but unfortunately this is not the case. In our busy lives, moms are lucky to grab a breakfast that contains something other than black coffee or a glass of juice. Then we continue the day by eating fast foods or convenience foods, which lack nutrients. Multi-vitamin supplements make sure we get all of our necessary vitamins and minerals. Without these essential nutrients you will not be able to see the fitness results you desire. If you are breastfeeding, you should continue taking your prenatal vitamin.

## Healthy Fats!

Essential Fatty Acids are the "good fats" that help un-do damage done to our bodies (hearts, arteries, veins) from the "bad fats" such as trans fats and cholesterol (animal fat). Good fats raise your HDL or "good cholesterol." High Density Lipoprotein (HDL) helps remove the "bad cholesterol", or LDL (Low Density Lipoprotein), by escorting it to the liver where it is broken down and excreted. This is very important in an age when so many of us are struggling to achieve and maintain healthy cholesterol levels, and fight heart disease and obesity.

## Water. It Really Is That Important!

The human body is more than 70% water. Without water, humans would die in a few days. Did you know a small 2% drop in your body's water supply can trigger signs of dehydration: headaches, tiredness and lack of focus!

An estimated 75% of Americans have mild, chronic dehydration. All cell and organ functions in our body depend on water. Water serves as a lubricant for joints and organs, regulates body temperature, alleviates constipation, and regulates metabolism. Drinking eight glasses of water daily can decrease the risk of colon cancer by 45%, bladder cancer by 50% and it can potentially even reduce the risk of breast cancer.

## *No Fad Diets*

Whether low-carb, low-calorie, or low-fat, it seems like there is always a marketing fueled gimmick to help you lose weight! We know moms wish there was that magic pill. So how many of these diets have you tried before?

- Low-carb diet
- Low-fat diet
- Liquid diet (using low-calorie, high-fiber shakes)
- Grapefruit diet
- Detox diet
- Cabbage Soup diet
- Macrobiotic diet
- The Juice diet

If you've followed at least one of these diets, you've had plenty of company. Problem is, if a diet really worked, we'd all be on it, and we'd stay on it! The reality is that fad diets don't help you lose the weight that stays off.

### *What is a Fad Diet?*

Fad diets promise quick weight loss in a very short time. The fact is, diets that sound too good to be true are!

*Tips to recognizing a fad diet*
- Most fad diets will restrict certain types of foods, while encouraging the dieter to eat another type of food.
- The diet makes claims that weight loss is quick and rapid, without the need to exercise. (Rapid weight loss is defined as anything greater than two pounds per week.)
- The diet promotes miracle foods that burn fat.
- The diet has a rigid menu with a list of foods that must be eaten at a specific time of the day or in specific combinations.
- The diet will not have a warning label.
- The diet will not have credible scientific research to back up its claims.
- Any diet that states absolute ratios of carbohydrates, proteins and fats. (For examples: 40, 30, 30 OR 60, 20, 20.)

Now we're going to let you know why these are not healthy post baby!

A side effect of fad diets is "yo-yo dieting." Yo-yo dieting is when a person goes on a diet, loses weight and then gains it back once they resume their normal way of eating. Frustrated with the weight gain, they try another diet. And the cycle continues. Research shows that people actually gain more overall weight with this type of dieting!

*Most common fad diets*

**Liquid Diets** – Most people who go on a liquid diet will probably lose weight. However, once the dieter resumes eating whole foods, the pounds pile back on. Liquid dieters are discouraged from being on a liquid diet for an extended period of time. That is because these diets do not provide the body with the proper amount of vitamins and minerals needed to maintain optimal health.

**High Protein Diets** – High protein diets claim that if you only eat large quantities of protein, you will lose fat and build muscle. However, high protein diets may cause damage to the liver and kidneys and must be balanced with whole grain carbohydrates, fruit, vegetables and healthy fats.

**Low-Fat Diets** – The body needs fat in order to burn fat. The theory behind low fat diets is to remove all fat, so that you will burn your own body fat. The problem is that the body does not work this way. Additionally, most low-fat foods add sugar to maintain taste! And sugar, as we know, is converted to blood sugar, which spikes our cravings and causes us to gain weight.

**One Food Diet (Example: Grapefruit Diet)** – This type of restrictive diet is very unhealthy and most people cannot maintain this type of diet. Weakness can occur quickly due to low calorie consumption, as well as a lack of vitamins and minerals in the food. In addition, the body will lower its metabolic rate and burn fewer calories.

## *ACSS's Favorite Healthy Food Choices*

*Starch Carbohydrates - necessary before and after hard workouts!*
- Oatmeal one-half cup - old fashioned, sweeten with sugar substitute and cinnamon
- Sweet or white potatoes 3-4 oz.
- Rice, any kind, one-half cup
- Cream of Wheat or Rice – read the package

- Cheerios or Total Cereal – 1 cup
- Ezekiel bread – 2 pieces

*Veggies: Serving is two cups raw, one cup cooked*
- Broccoli
- Asparagus
- Green beans
- Sugar snap peas
- Spinach, green leaf lettuce
- Salad fixing veggies
- Peppers (red, yellow, green)
- Cauliflower

*Fruits: Serving is whole fruit – medium sized*
- Grapefruit
- Pineapple
- Apple
- Peach
- Pear
- Berries (strawberry, blueberry, raspberry, blackberry) – one-quarter cup

*Protein: The ideal serving is 4-6 oz. per meal (1 oz. = 7 grams of protein)*
- Chicken
- Fish – tuna, any white fish, salmon *on occasion*
- Turkey
- Egg whites
- Low-carb, low-fat protein powder – 1 scoop
- Lean red meat – tenderloin, 98% ground beef, flank – grilled, so fat drips off
- Dairy – low-fat/non-fat cheese, not-fat yogurt, skim milk, low-fat cottage cheese

*Fats:*
- Flax
- Olive oil to cook with
- Almonds, cashews, walnuts

*Sweets / Snacks:*

- Sugar free pudding or Jell-O
- Sugar free popsicles

*Drinks:*
- Water (minimum 8 glasses a day)
- Sugar free Kool-aid, Crystal Light, iced tea
- Coffee (watch what you add into this)

# *Protein, a Building Block for Good Nutrition*

Learn how to use it in your cooking! Many people wonder if they can actually cook with protein. The answer is yes. Heat *denatures* proteins, which means it changes the shape of the protein molecules. For example, in the case of cooking eggs, the texture of the egg changes from liquid to firm. In the same way, cooking changes the shape of the protein in powders, but will leave the amino acids found in those proteins intact as long as the oven temperature does not exceed 400 degrees. Cooking at lower temperatures may require slightly increased cooking times, but the finished product is so worth it!

Many people replace some of the flour in traditional recipes with protein powder. Remember, protein cannot be substituted cup for cup. Think of it as "glue" for all the other ingredients. It contains no gluten, so it will not rise like flour, so you will need to adjust accordingly by adding baking powder and baking soda. Only replace half of the flour with protein powder, and leave the rest of the flour in. The texture can become rubbery if too much protein powder is added, so use caution when adding protein so as not to remove all of the fats. Another important consideration is the flavor you want to add, as chocolate may not taste so great for breakfast.

*Great Protein Recipes from ACSS*

### Oatmeal (one serving)

Cook your normal serving of regular oatmeal and add half to one scoop of any flavor of protein powder for a powered breakfast of protein and whole grain carbohydrates to fuel your morning.

### Protein Pancakes (make a batch of pancakes: 15 small or 8 big)
- 4 egg whites
- 1 1/4 cup skim milk – Blend these first and then add dry ingredients

- 4 scoops of healthy heart Bisquick (use the protein scoop to measure this)
- 2 scoops of protein – (add one scoop at a time and keep blending)

Options for other tasty ingredients...

Chopped walnuts, almonds or pecans with banana protein powder

Blueberries (add in after all blended)

Crushed flaxseed

### Pancakes – On the leaner side (one serving)
- 4 egg whites
- 1/2 cup oatmeal
- 1/2 scoop protein powder
- 1 tsp. of baking powder
- 1-2 packets of sugar substitute
- Mix the above, spray pan and cook as normal, serve with spray butter and sugar-free syrup

### Sweet Potato Pancakes (one serving)
- 3 ounces cooked sweet potato
- 3 egg whites
- 1 scoop protein powder
- 1 packet of sugar substitute
- 1 tsp. baking powder
- Pumpkin Pie spice mix to taste

For best taste and texture blend all of the above ingredients in a mixer or blender and then cook as a pancake.

### Cookies, Brownies, Muffins, or Cakes

You can add protein to almost any recipe. Start by replacing one to two scoops of your flour or box mix with the same amount of chocolate, cappuccino, vanilla, or banana protein powder (or other flavor of your choice). Make sure you do not set the oven for a temperature higher than 350 degrees or your baked goods will burn as the protein is denatured; this requires longer cook times and keeping a close eye. Keep the cooking temperature at 350 degrees or lower. This may require longer cooking times.

**Pumpkin Pie**

Follow the regular recipe but replace the condensed milk with non-fat condensed milk, the sugar with sugar substitute, and add in one to two scoops of vanilla protein powder.

**Caffeine and Protein**

Add one or two scoops of chocolate protein powder to black coffee for a low-fat, low-sugar café mocha. Or try vanilla protein powder and skim milk for that great vanilla latte taste.

## ACSS Team's Recommended Cookbooks for New Moms

We promise these recipes from are tried and true cookbooks are easy and most are kid approved!
- *The Eat Clean Diet Cookbook* by Tosco Reno
- *Cook Yourself Thin & Cook Yourself Thin Faster* – These recipes are on the smaller portion side, so if you are sharing with the family or significant other, double the portion! Favorites – Spaghetti and Meatballs, Turkey Chili, Sweet Potato Fries.
- *Cook This Not That* – This is the cookbook that teaches you how to cook all your restaurant favorites. And wait until you see the difference in calories!

# Exercise (Mom & Baby)

Once you get the thumbs up from your healthcare provider to begin exercising, the key is to start slowly, and gradually increase the duration of exercise and your intensity!

The ACSS Transitions Team uses the baby's age as a scale for how intense the mom's exercise should be.
- **0-3 months** – Do exercises similar to the third trimester of pregnancy
- **4-6 months** – Exercises similar to the second trimester
- **7 months on** – Most moms can return to the majority of their exercises with some small changes (all based on the individual)

## How Do I Find the Time to Exercise?

Sometimes the most meaningful and most convenient way to exercise is to incorporate your baby into your new exercise routine. You can walk with a stroller or while wearing your baby in a carrier. On days when the weather is inclement, head to the local mall. Additionally, there are some facilities that offer exercise classes that allow you to bring your baby with you – look for the key words "Mommy and Me" in the description. However, these classes are most appropriate for babies two months old to age one or two years.

Naptime can be an opportunity to exercise, but women often look at the dishes, the laundry or other chores and feel that they need to postpone exercising. Then suddenly naptime is over! If this is the case for you, try setting a limit on cleaning time. Do as much as you can in 10 or 15 minutes and leave the rest for later. Give yourself 20 minutes to exercise and go from there. Maybe some days you will exercise longer, or some days you will start the next load of laundry. Either way, you will feel better at everything you need to do when you are taking time to care for yourself and your body.

---

### Go for a Walk

Do not feel bad about asking someone to watch the baby so you can have alone time to go for a walk. This time apart is beneficial for both Mom and Baby, especially if dad or family is watching the baby! Your time is critical for healing and feeling good about your new body!

---

## Pre-Pregnancy Weight

This depends on how much weight you gained during pregnancy, your metabolism, level of physical activity and whether you are breastfeeding. Breastfeeding uses almost one-third of our caloric intake. Postpartum is not a time for dieting. Instead, by eating a variety of whole foods and drinking at least three liters of water per day, you can help your body to self-regulate. When we combine a healthy diet with regular physical activity such as walking, swimming, yoga or even cleaning the house, we release the weight of pregnancy.

## *Am I Doing Too Much?*

A sure sign that you are too aggressive with your postpartum exercise is if your vaginal discharge, or lochia, turns bright pink or red. If you notice any changes, slow down. Notify your healthcare provider if your lochia starts again after it has tapered off.

*Note: it is normal for your lochia to increase slightly with activity – a color change to bright red is the best indicator of new bleeding and an indication that you are doing too much.*

The important thing to remember is to be gentle with yourself and follow your healthcare provider's advice. Make sure you're eating a healthy diet, particularly if you're breastfeeding. Stay well-hydrated and don't give up. Fitting in exercise may be hit or miss as you adjust to your new life and baby. So do the best you can and focus your energy on taking care of yourself and your baby.

## *Does Postpartum Exercise Decrease Milk Production?*

No – and it has no adverse effect on the baby. In a study at the University of North Carolina at Greensboro, where 40 overweight lactating women were assigned to either a diet and exercise group or a control group for 10 weeks, there was no significant difference between groups in terms of milk produced for their infants. The new mothers in the exercise group did indeed see a weight loss.

## *Is it True that I Shouldn't Exercise Before Breastfeeding?*

Some studies have shown that lactic acid build up in Mom can slightly alter the taste of breast milk, causing some infants to reject it. However everything returns to normal after an hour or so. To avoid this, you may want to feed your baby or pump a half-hour before you exercise. Your breasts will also be less heavy and your baby will be less likely to interrupt your workout due to hunger.

## *Sample Postpartum Workout*

| Where | Example Exercises |
|---|---|
| *With Baby* | **Pushups with baby**<br>These are regular knee pushups, with baby lying beneath mommy looking up at her.<br><br>**Crunches with baby**<br>Hold baby on mom's knees and make funny faces every time you come up. |
| *Stairs and Baby Carrier* | **Up and down**<br>Carrying baby in carrier, walk up and down your flight of stairs in your house. Be sure to the use the hand railing.<br><br>**Squats**<br>Holding baby, sit on couch, then stand up, and repeat for repetitions. |
| *Stroller Outside* | **Walking**<br>This old standby has been used by generations of moms and is still one of the easiest ways to get some quick exercise.<br><br>**Lunges behind stroller**<br>These are typical walking lunges, just do it while pushing the stroller.<br><br>**Pushups using stroller**<br>Put your hands on the handlebar, and push up and down, again making funny faces at baby (make sure the stroller is in locked position)! |

Table 6. Sample Postpartum Workout.

# Stress Management

## *Focus on Being Positive*

As mothers, we know how important it is to focus on the positives, especially at this time when life can be exceptionally stressful. Positive thinking provided us with a way to stay even-keeled, upbeat and joyful, even in times of difficulty or crisis, and allowed for continued enjoyment of life. Learning how to be positive can have a lasting impact on your daily life so make it a point to use it.

Here are some of the positive thinking techniques we used and now share with other moms to help enjoy this journey called motherhood:

**Smile** – One easy way to stay positive is to smile. Smiling helps the immune system to work better. Smiling has been shown to increase immune function and helps you feel more relaxed. Even if you are feeling down or overwhelmed, smile! Why? Smiling can help trick your body into helping you change your mood. Another great benefit of smiling is the release endorphins, natural pain killers, and serotonin. These three chemicals will give you a natural high!

**Prioritize** – Know what is important and take care of that first. Don't feel the pressure to push and take care of everything. It's unrealistic and a huge stressor. As moms, we must learn to prioritize. For instance, if a mom desperately wants to find the time to exercise and eat right for weight loss after pregnancy, but that task seems impossible with her baby demanding every moment of every day, how can she find the time and motivation to lose weight? This is the time to prioritize. Take a few moments when your baby is sleeping and plan on how to make some nutritional meals and snacks ahead of time. Also, write down an exercise plan that factors in your baby's patterns. Whether it is a 10 or 15 minute walk with your baby in a stroller, or finding a gym that provides childcare to assist you in meeting your goals, you will be on your way to a healthier and happier you!

**Delegating** – Some moms feel very uncomfortable passing along tasks even though others can take care of them. Don't feel like it is all up to you! Delegating tasks whenever possible is a great way to take some pressure off and help others feel like a bigger part of family life after baby's arrival. Your husband/partner can be a great resource in helping things run smoothly. If you have older children, this is a great way to help them learn responsibility and give you a welcome break. For some women, giving up control can seem difficult to do, but really it helps gain back control of your life.

**Saying No** – You have a lot less personal and social time than you did before the baby. It's okay to pick and choose the activities or invitations which are important to you. Some moms push themselves to make everyone happy. Others don't feel comfortable saying "no". Not only is it okay, but it can be very necessary for reducing stress and maintaining a balance in your life.

**Meditation** – Practicing meditation naturally calms the mind and relaxes the body. It is conscious relaxation and an extremely effective way to increase focus and address the problems that you may be dealing with. Sit quietly for 10 to 30 minutes in the morning or evening. This will give your mind and body time to relax and relieve tension. Note how negativity and tension disappear as you meditate. Just concentrating on your breathing will put you in a positive state of mind. The more you meditate the more positive thinking will become a natural part of your consciousness. Take the time to learn about meditation and incorporate it into your life. Your body and mind will thank you! For those who feel they just can't meditate – try listening to your favorite music. This will instantly make you positive because music that you like has been shown raise your mood.

**Affirmations** – Affirmations are a great positive thinking technique. Regular use of affirmations reinforces positive thinking and can overcome the effects of previously held bad attitudes. It is surprisingly easy and can be done almost anywhere. An affirmation is a statement of declaration that reinforces or affirms a strong belief. It is important to understand that a positive affirmation statement is a firm and passionate declaration. You can use "I am" to begin your affirmation and make sure it is a positive statement such as, "I am a happy and positive person." All you need to do is recite your affirmation daily as often as you like but at least several times a day. It is good to make it a habit to do a positive affirmation at a fixed time everyday and then whenever you need it.

**Journaling** – Another positive thinking activity is journaling. Putting your thoughts down on paper is a very good therapeutic activity. Journaling changes your perspective by cathartically releasing emotions or concerns that you've kept pent up inside. This will allow you to look at things with a little more perspective and, for many, makes decisions easier. By looking at an issue from a different standpoint once it's on paper, it is often easier to see a positive solution.

**Stay in the present and savor right now** – One way to alleviate stress is to appreciate the moment. Try to stay in the moment rather than always thinking about the past or the future. Be in the present, relax, and find happiness in where you are right now. Enjoy where you and your baby are right now. Cherish his or her smile, and this time in your lives that you are sharing together. Take just ten seconds and "breathe" in the moment. Be fully engrossed by what your senses are taking in.

**Go slow** – Just like making a choice to stay in the moment, making a conscious choice to take life more slowly will empower you to enjoy the little snuggles with your baby in the morning without feeling rushed to start your day. These precious little moments with your baby will go so fast, so don't miss a minute of it!

**Reward yourself** – Now that you're regaining control of your life, do something for yourself as a reward for handling the obstacles. Now is your chance to finish that book you started reading, or the art project you didn't have time to start. Maybe you would enjoy trying a new restaurant or a walk in the park. Perhaps you just want to lie on the couch and watch a movie. Go ahead, enjoy yourself. You've earned it. You deserve it!

# Conclusion

Take care of your health, your mind and your body. When you are healthy, you look and feel great. It is important to give your body what it needs. Make sure you are making healthy food choices and take recommended supplements as needed. What we feed our bodies does determine in large measure how we handle the effects of emotional stress.

# Moving Beyond 9 Months

Congrats, Mom! You are moving into a new phase of motherhood and also in your workout routine. Not only is your body healing nicely, but your baby is on the move too!

ACSS has worked with hundreds of postnatal moms and the most common complaint from 7-12 months postnatal is, "Why haven't I lost all my baby weight – yet?" It takes time, so please be patient with yourself. Whatever the reason, if you still haven't reached your goal weight, don't feel bad. Fifty percent of moms don't get back to "pre-baby" shape until the one year mark, and twenty percent don't get there until the two year mark! It really is all about balance! In addition to adding in regular weight training, now is the time to add in plyometrics – exercises that require agility, strength and power, and in the end strengthen ligaments and tendons.

Bonus, you can still find time to workout being a full time mom and a career woman. It's get in, get moving, get out and back to the hectic pace of life. Because of this need, Corry created a Boot Camp For Moms class. One mom commented, "Just six weeks after having my first child I was ready to hit the gym and Boot Camp For Moms seemed perfect for me. The program helped me transition back into a regular exercise routine by teaching me the correct and safe way to work out postpartum. Certain exercises were modified for me so that I was able to do each work out safely and also effectively. It's also encouraging to have other moms who are, or have been, in similar circumstances there to motivate you to reach your fitness goals."

Read more reviews of Boot Camp For Moms on the Nine Months In Nine Months Out website at (www.9monthsin9monthsout.com).

Boot camp participants range from the new mom of six months, to moms with several children, and fit moms just looking to get their focus back. Corry modifies the exercises as needed based on how recently a mother has given birth. "The body goes through many stages and while jumping isn't ok two to three months postpartum, it gets shapely results when the time is right, where moms need it most – our butt and thighs!"

## *The Ultimate Boot Camp For Moms Workout*

*No equipment necessary*

- Walking lunges 3 x 30
  - ~ Superset with 3 x 10 regular pushups
- Diagonal walking lunges 3 x 30
  - ~ Superset with 3 x 15 triceps pushups
- Walking "pump" lunges
  - ~ Superset with 3 x 20 Pop squats
- Plank with one arm rows 4 x 10 (pushup/balance variation for the back)
  - ~ Superset with 3 x 50 crunches

**Walking lunge** – Take a big step forward and bend both knees to a right angle. Then step the back leg in and through without touching the floor so you are in the next lunge. Each rep coincides with one leg, so 3 x 30 is 3 sets of 30 lunges. Variations to the walking lunge really get the burn and hit what most women call their "trouble spots" regardless if they have had a baby or not. The diagonal lunge takes a lateral, or step, to the right side to target the inner/outer thigh. Just as you are bending into the lunge turn the back or left leg to line both set of toes facing forward. On coming up, turn to the left, stepping left (about a 45 degree angle) and then twist body in and continue. The pumping lunge is the same as the regular walking lunge except you step into the lunge, pump up to almost straight legs, then down and step forward.

**Regular Pushups** – Make sure hands are wider than the shoulders and body is in a plank position (hips are in a straight line with heels, shoulders and head). Slowly lower the body to the ground, elbows stay directly above the wrists, exhale and push the body back up to the plank. If using the knee option place both the knees and the feet on the ground and keep the hips level with the rest of the body.

**Tricep Pushups** – Same plank motion but the hands are directly in line with the shoulders. Bend the elbows backward keeping them touching the sides of the body, exhale and push back up. Knee option is the same here.

**One arm rows** – In plank position used for either exercise above, lift one hand up without rotating the spine and then place back down. Lift the other hand and repeat for total reps.

**Pop squats** – Start standing with legs together, jump legs out into a squat (knees stay in line with toes, buttocks back, abs in) then jump back in squeezing inner thighs together, into a standing upright position. Repeat – this is a plyometric move that strengthens the ligaments and tendons.

# Stress Management

Hopefully, by now, you've worked out a household routine. Maybe you're up with your baby, getting him/her fed, then settling them down in the swing while you change the laundry and dishes around. A few minutes later, you're able to sit down with breakfast and a strong cup of tea.

*Your stress management goals going forward include:*
- Establish a routine – Make sure you have a morning routine that sets you up for success for the rest of the day.
- Making time to exercise – Movement can make all the difference in your day, get those endorphins flowing.
- Eating right – It benefits you and your baby!
- Scheduling time for you – Whether it's a few minutes to steal away and take a hot bath, write in your journal, or simply breathe, we all still need a little 'me' time during our day.

You're doing a great job! We all learn as we go along. Surround yourself with positive people and thoughts; it will naturally lift up your mood.

# Parental Skills

We all learned certain parenting skills from watching our parents and experiencing childhood ourselves. Now it's time to experience parenthood, and we get to decide for ourselves what kind of parents we want to be.

You're likely dealing with the thoughts of going back to work, or staying at home and make adjustments to your household living standards. These are challenging decisions.

For some mothers, now is the time to figure out how to cope with being away from your baby for hours at a time.

Finding the right quality and affordable childcare solution is critically important. For research tips to help research the right childcare solution for you, check out www.9monthsin9monthsout.com.

*Some ways to ease back into the work force:*
- Check with your supervisor and start back part time.
- Start out with the day care provider part time before going back to work, so you know you can be there in moments if you need to be.
- Can some of your work be done from home? If so, start back one or two days a week while your child is in day care.

It takes a unique focus to be able to work with your baby around; try to learn to balance and realize that your baby is going to love playing and interacting with other babies!

# The Birth Stories

## A Birth Story: Angel J. Miller

When my husband Randy and I decided to have a baby, we had been married almost four years. I was told by my ob/gyn if I did get pregnant, I would be considered a "high risk" pregnancy because I had recently been diagnosed with an "incompetent cervix." I come from the generation of daughters whose mothers were given a drug called DES to prevent miscarriages back in the day (1950's to early 1970's). This drug is well known for causing fertility issues with the offspring and also malformed reproductive organs.

After three months of trying, I was pregnant! This all occurred before entering nursing school and midwifery school so I had a lot of questions and concerns because of my high risk status and what to expect because of this status. My doctor at that time was considered a high risk specialist and I was to have a cerclage placed at 14 weeks (a stitch that holds the cervix closed) and have prenatal visits every two weeks after my surgery until 36 weeks, then weekly. I did not ask any questions, just followed everything I was told to do. I was working full time and was on my feet a lot. I gained too much weight (55 pounds) and paid for it in the end. At 35 weeks, I developed mild pre-eclampsia and was put on bed rest. At 36 weeks and on Mother's Day Weekend, while my husband was painting baby furniture in the garage and I was "nesting", my water broke! I was scared because having the cerclage, I knew I had to go into the hospital right away. I was not mentally ready for this! I called the emergency number and found out my physician was not on call. I spoke with a physician I had never met, but he seemed kind and re-assuring. He advised me to come in right away. Again, this was Mother's Day weekend and it was Saturday, not a good window of opportunity for personal hospitality services in any hospital. After cleaning up, we made our way to the hospital and I was having irregular contractions.

When we arrived, the labor and delivery unit was busy so I was escorted to a labor room across from the operating room (OR). I had to have my cerclage removed before anything else could be done. I was placed on the fetal monitor to monitor my baby's heartbeat and the few contractions I was having, prepped for surgery (IV, epidural), and the cerclage was easily removed. I immediately dilated to 4 cm when the cerclage was removed and I was excited! I thought "I am already 4 cm without having any contractions!!" Little did I know it was going to be a very long, drawn out and complicated process during a holiday weekend.

After my water had been broken for 29 hours and after 18 hours of painful contractions with Pitocin, my cervix never changed! I handled them pretty well with Randy's help, but was exhausted, and my husband was exhausted. I developed a high fever and the baby's heart rate was increasing. I had gone through three shifts of nurses and the physician on call on this Mother's Day was not very patient with anyone. He was very abrupt and just kept increasing the Pitocin without any explanation. He did scare us with the fact that since the baby is only 36 weeks, he would probably be whisked away to the ICU and placed in an incubator because he would be small, and I wouldn't be able to hold him. My husband asked him how long he would proceed with the Pitocin since I had developed a fever, and the doctor informed him we would have to proceed with a cesarean section since I had a fever and it was putting our baby at risk. My husband needed to run home quickly to take care of our Siberian Husky Misha who had been alone since we came to the hospital. There was no one else to take care of her. The doctor re-assured my husband he would turn off the Pitocin and proceed to a C/S within the hour. My husband was my rock during those painful contractions, and when he left, the nurse continued to turn up the Pitocin. I was unprepared for this, and being exhausted and by myself, I just began to sob. The nurse was very curt to me and non-supportive, bluntly telling me to stop crying and deal with it. It was obvious she did not want to be working during this time. As a side bar, epidurals at this time were not on a continuous pump, they had to be re-dosed each time. They would let the epidural dose totally wear off before re-dosing. Anesthesia was very busy (short staff) that day and could not come out of the operating room (OR) to re-dose the epidural which had not been re-dosed since that morning when the Pitocin was started. By the time Randy came back (the longest hour in my life) I was hysterically crying. Randy was not happy and wanted to speak with the physician. After a quiet one on one with the physician, we proceeded to the OR for the birth of our son on Mother's Day. What a wonderful present! He came out unscathed, with a good strong cry and weighed 7 pounds 9 ounces at 36 weeks! Two units of blood later, I was in the recovery room holding my son. Shea Michal Miller was absolutely beautiful!

I developed a severe infection (endometritis) and was on triple antibiotics and in the hospital for the next six days. It was rough, but it was worth it and I would have done it again. Unfortunately, Mother Nature had other plans for me, and I was unable to conceive after several years of trying and going through infertility work-up and treatments.

At first I was angry, then very sad that I could not conceive again, enduring test after test on myself and on my husband. Nothing was found to be wrong, which I guess was a good thing, but we were never able to conceive again.

My son is now a 28 year old healthy young man whom I am very proud of! As a nurse midwife I get to birth and hold new babies every week which is an ongoing lovely satisfaction my life.

# A Birth Story: Corry L. Matthews

I always knew I wanted to be a mommy; I just wasn't sure when that day would come. When the time came that I knew I wanted to be a mom, I wanted to be pregnant that very day, and let's just say, I am not the most patient person. After being married almost nine years, my husband and I decided we would stop preventing pregnancy and start trying… assuming it would take a few months to a year. The second month, with the help of an ovulation predictor kit, I was pregnant! I actually took two tests just to be sure!

Morning sickness, well, in my case it was all day sickness, sunk in at about five weeks, and lasted until fourteen weeks. I remember one evening lying on the couch feeling horrible and reminding myself how excited I was to meet this amazing new life growing inside of me… I could do this. During the first trimester my food choices consisted of: hotdogs (yuck, I know), Spagettios (they are toddler food, must be sort of nutritious), saltines, and ginger anything. Forget about any type of protein, breakfast that used to be oatmeal and egg whites was now plain white bagels… any type of complex carbs brought on more nausea! The first trimester workouts consisted of lifting three days per week legs/shoulders, back/bis, chest/tris (which I did in under 30 minutes) and mainly walking, about 30 minutes, 40 if the morning sickness stayed away. I tried to do my group exercise classes but spent more time throwing up than enjoying the class! My initial starting weight was 142 pounds (I gained about seven from December after my last show until I found out I was pregnant – and began adding more carbohydrates to prepare my body for the marathon of pregnancy).

They give you so much information at the doctor's office. Unfortunately for the *worrying me*, the fact that stuck in my head was the one about miscarriage and how more than 15% of all pregnancies will end in miscarriage. This percent decreases to about 5% once you hear the heart beat, so my first ultrasound at nine weeks was so amazing! The sound of that little heartbeat will forever stay etched in my memory! At 12 weeks we did the first trimester screening – and everything turned out perfectly normal! I was amazed at how much the baby grew in three weeks! For me the ultrasounds and doctor's appointments were the most re-assuring moments of pregnancy in those first few months when I couldn't feel the baby moving.

When I reached about 14 weeks I went through the "Am I really still pregnant? I feel so good" stage. Well, feeling good was relative based on what I had been feeling. I felt a burst of energy and a renewed sense for wanting to get back into the gym – and work harder. I returned to my Body Step classes and did weight training three days per week – same types of exercises, just different intensity now that I was pregnant. Instead of pop squats I did wide leg squats, instead of walking lunges, I did stationary lunges – but overall I felt great. By my 4th and 5th month the belly was looking more like a baby belly and not a "is she still working out?" belly. At 18 weeks we had the anatomy ultrasound, and I was so nervous. My husband and I wanted to know the sex of the baby, but wanted to keep it a secret from everyone else until the baby arrived. I was really hoping for a little girl, and when they told us it was a she and not a he, I was grinning from ear to ear.

My pregnancy progressed beautifully without complications. I was right on schedule – the schedule I knew I would maintain, of gaining one pound a week (without shoes of course). I continued with my group exercise classes and walking right up until Alex was born. In the 2nd and 3rd trimesters I was lucky and unlucky that my appetite came back. The good news was I could enjoy my protein shakes and egg whites again; the bad news was I had intense cravings for Taco Bell and McDonald's! I walked the dogs every morning, and it soon became very apparent to all my neighbors that the coat and belly were getting bigger and bigger.

January 7th, her due date came and went. I was 50% effaced since 36 weeks but nothing was changing. At 40 weeks they told me they were scheduling my induction for the following week so I got on the phone with my acupuncturist to see how we could make this little girl come on her own - naturally. Well, she is stubborn (just like her mom) and we went to the hospital on January 12th, 2009 for the induction. I was so nervous on the way to the hospital, and of course there was traffic living in Washington, D.C. My husband told me to put music in to calm my mind – Body Step it was, something about it allowed my mind to stop racing.

Once in the labor room a dear friend and certified nurse midwife, Angel, greeted me. She knew my birth plan was written for a completely natural birth, but when you start with Cervidil to get the cervix to open and dilate that is often hard. We choose the Cervidil since her head was down, but not on my cervix. After about two hours we had to remove the medicine as I had a major allergic reaction. We waited about two hours and then began the Pitocin. Even after 13 hours of Pitocin I was only 80% effaced and not even 1 cm dilated. Around 10pm the nurse came in and told me to get in the bed and lie on my left side and that we were cutting off the Pitocin.

The baby's heart rate was elevated yet her movement was down. In addition, my temperature was rising. We actually changed rooms because our room had become too hot. Around 11:45p the doctor said she wanted to watch me and the baby for 30 minutes and if things did not look better they wanted to do a c-section. What did I do…CRIED! I was worried about this precious little baby. I was so thankful for having both my husband and good friend Vickie by my side at this point. About six weeks prior to her birth I began reading the Hypnobirth book nightly and did the meditation daily. And although my birth plan went from natural, to induction drugs, to spinal anesthesia, to a c-section, I remained calm the entire time, knowing the end result was always healthy Mom and healthy Baby.

Alexandra Noelle Matthews was born at 1:24am on January 13th. I got to breastfeed her in the post delivery room before she headed off with daddy for a bath and measurements.

We spent about four days in the hospital. I knew a c-section was major surgery but I assumed since I was really fit I would be different. I was shocked at how hard it was to get out of bed, or to pick Alex up out of her crib. If there was a side effect I had it: itching from the spinal, gas pains from the c-section, fears of blood clots with varicose veins, cracked and bleeding nipples! Having a baby hurts – but is SO VERY worth it!

The first couple of weeks were rough adjusting to the new baby. I began feeling depressed as soon as we got home – but wasn't really sure why. The first day home I cried because I was afraid she was going to grow up too fast! The depression continued when at five weeks I learned that Alex's sucking had not been enough to maintain my milk supply and since she was eating every hour I wasn't pumping and did not realize my milk had disappeared. We ended up in the emergency room because she was dehydrated.

At that point I worked daily with a board certified La Leche League coach and we tried everything: drugs (whose side effect for me was further depression), hospital grade pumps, herbal supplements (Mother's Milk – More Milk Plus), syringes with formula in them and nothing would bring my milk supply back.

At eight weeks I decided it was time to switch to formula; nursing for 20 minutes, pumping for 15 minutes and then giving her a bottle, which was repeated 45 minutes after finishing wasn't working. She still wasn't gaining enough weight and I knew teaching her to only suck from a bottle was best for her and for me. I could say I cried over all of it, *but that would be lying* – I laid in bed bawling over not being able to breastfeed my daughter. I went over every single "what if I had done this, or that". Once I had grieved not being able to feed her, then came the feelings of regret and upset over not being able to lose the baby weight with breastfeeding as well. So next time you see a mom giving her baby a bottle, before you jump in and ask "why aren't you breastfeeding" remember there may be a very painful story associated with the why!

Celebrating Alex turning one!

It is a bittersweet moment to watch your little baby graduate from just that, being a baby, and move on to toddlerhood! She is walking and saying "momma" and "hi" and changes every single day! It took me a total of 40 weeks to lose all of my baby weight, and I am so happy to say that I took all of that time to do it. The best part, I feel better than I have ever felt in my entire life. I have a new sense of appreciation for my healthy body, and the image I used to see in the mirror that I thought needed this toned or that smaller…well, I now love that image and could not be happier.

I get asked all the time what my nutrition looks like as a mom on the go… in addition to being a mom, I own a Sports Nutrition store, am a Regional Director for the Max Muscle franchise in VA, chair the Health and Wellness Business Council for PW County, serve as the President for Fit & Healthy Schools, and conduct Boot Camps For Moms and prenatal personal training. It is a lot, but I love what I do!

*Here it is…*

- Pre –Workout, first meal of the day: Maxpro Protein with skim milk, English muffin with Smart Balance Butter
- Post-Workout: Iso-Extreme protein shake mixed with water and XTR (glutamine blend) and ½ cup of oatmeal.
- Lunch (1 or 2pm): Carbs, protein and veggies (or if I can't get the veggies in Green Synergy)
- 5pm: Another shake
- 7:30pm: Dinner – and it is whatever I cook for my family!

Having Alex is the best thing I have ever done! With all my certifications, degrees, and titles I knew the one I was missing was "MOM"!

# A Birth Story: Shelia L. Kirkbride

I can't totally put into words the excitement I felt when I found out I was pregnant. It had only been about eight weeks before when I had a miscarriage. My miscarriage had been very devastating and so unexpected. Excitement turned to sadness very quickly.

Being pregnant again brought some real fear this time, a kind I hadn't experienced before, along with wonderful joy and excitement. I really wanted to be a mom and was so scared something might go wrong again. Happily my pregnancy did progress along. Unfortunately, the morning sickness began. I don't know why it's called morning sickness because for me it lasted all day long. Wow! Those hormones work a number on the body.

My pregnancy was one of the happiest times in my life, but at the same time, one of the most difficult emotionally and physically. While I was pregnant my father passed away so this time was bitter sweet. My husband was in the military and completing Officer Candidate School in Quantico, Virginia, so I had chosen to stay with my family and spend some time with them. Unfortunately, I was only there two weeks when he died. I was dealing with grief, the physical changes in my body, and all day "morning sickness".

When I was in my second trimester I moved to Quantico while my husband continued training. It was nice being in Virginia and connecting with other spouses. Quite a few were pregnant and it was nice to commiserate. Their friendship and support meant so much!

After my husband's graduation from OCS we moved together to Marine Corps Base Quantico, Virginia while he completed training at The Basic School. It was nice because I connected with several women whose husbands were also going through training. Quite a few were even pregnant and it was nice to commiserate. Their friendship and support meant so much.

In true military style, my son Joshua would arrive by cesarean while his father was involved in a military training exercise which was called the "Nine Day War". I physically and emotionally felt like I had just participated in a nine day war myself. I had been scheduled for a cesarean section that morning, but when I arrived at the hospital they decided to induce.

So for twelve hours I was hooked up to Pitocin. Unfortunately, I never dilated more than a couple of centimeters and my physician suggested we go with the cesarean now. So around seven o'clock Joshua would arrive. I was so thankful he was healthy and had no abnormalities. But Josh had swallowed some meconium and he was being monitored. Josh was two weeks late and he had suffered some stress. At least this was what the doctored believed had happened.

Recovering from the cesarean was difficult. I was very fatigued almost all of the time. I would walk into a store from my car weeks after the birth and still feel like I needed to sit down. Trying to take care of Josh and myself would be a challenge. My energy was definitely going to take a while to return. Luckily I would have visits from both grandmothers which were a blessing. Unfortunately, fatigue would not be the only thing I would have to deal with.

I didn't know about the baby blues, and I definitely wasn't aware of something called postpartum depression after I had my son. This statement might be very surprising combined with the fact my mom was a nurse with an ob/gyn practice for over 20 years. She had flown threw her pregnancy with me and into motherhood without skipping a beat; she even worked the day she had me and walked to the hospital on her lunch hour to check herself in. She would never suffer from the baby blues or postpartum after she delivered me. She went into motherhood with a joy and excitement I could only have dreamt of.

Mine would be very different. I would understand how it feels. I am one of those women who suffered from anxiety and depression, so severe at times, the world appeared a scary place; I wondered how my child and I could make it through safely day to day. Not every woman who suffered from postpartum deals with the same issues but the connecting factors are the escalated level of anxiety and depression along with the difficulty experienced in dealing with daily life.

There was a lack of being educated about what would and could happen after delivery. My doctor did not ask how I was emotionally feeling after delivery as he did about my physical health. You could say I never saw it coming. No game plan was in place with coping techniques and no true understanding that it wasn't my fault for being what I considered "inadequate".

One of the scariest parts of postpartum can be the awareness something is wrong but not knowing what to do and blaming yourself for not "feeling" the way you should. I did feel there must be something wrong with me. I knew others who had babies recently and seemed, from my vantage point, to move effortlessly into the role of motherhood. So it must be me having a problem adjusting to motherhood.

Education for moms is so important! I also want moms to know they are never alone. If you can be educated and supported through pregnancy and beyond then motherhood can be enjoyed for the blessing it is!

## A Birth Story: Dr. Stacia D. Kelly

My mother went through seven miscarriages to have me. Knowing this, I spent two years preparing myself mentally and physically to even attempt to carry a baby once I'd felt ready to care for one. I read everything I could about healthy eating, learned about working out in the gym, and made slow but steady changes in the household fitness and nutrition processes.

Some women out there are blessed. They get and stay pregnant at the drop of a hat. Others are more challenged and try for years, some with success, some without.

After two years of trying I'd given up. I wasn't interested in doing in vitro. It's a great option for many, but I didn't want to chance the multiples or the disappointment. I figured, eventually, if I really felt the need to be a mom, there was adoption. There are so many children out there in need of a good and loving family.

And, then, I found out a week or so later, I was pregnant.

Excitement, yet certain calmness settled over me. I started reading everything I could. A few books that shall remain nameless scared the hell out of me. I kept up my workouts, slept when I needed to and started playing a nightly meditation CD that I used throughout my pregnancy.

Years and years before, I'd seen a show on the Discovery channel that showcased Hypnobirthing® and I thought, if I was ever going to have a baby, that was the way I was going to do it, calmly and without pain. Our society is so focused on pain and timing; we forget that women have been birthing babies forever and then going right back to what they were doing.

Because I'd been eating well and taking my vitamins, I had very few cravings (we're not counting the late night my husband so valiantly went out to get me a 3 Musketeers bar and cracked his tailbone and his wrist on the ice from sliding down our front stairs). I did get nauseous and dizzy a few times, but I really tried to pay attention to what my body needed and kept myself moving as much as possible. I might have weighed 116lbs when I found out I was pregnant. I think I gained 36lbs total. I kept a very careful chart. I read everything I could and slowly learned to ignore the horror stories. I'd even catch my friends in mid sentence if they were starting down a path of 'oh, it was just so hard…" I didn't want to hear it. And even more importantly, for me, I didn't want the baby hearing it. My family and those close to me learned quickly and would cut people off before they could even get started.

I knew I was having a boy (my poor mother kept telling me it was a girl, sorry Mom!). The ultrasound only confirmed it. We'd picked out a name when we were just dating, playing the 'what-if' game. Those first pictures still make me smile. I'm a writer, a creative, and here we'd created the ultimate…this tiny life that we were now responsible for. Scary, it took my husband a long time to catch up with my happiness and contentment. (You ask him now and he completely agrees that our son is the best thing ever!)

Healthy foods, constant walking, weight lifting with my trainer who was a few weeks further along than I was… all these things kept me motivated and focused. The scare came when the ob/gyn kept sending me back for ultrasounds. Our little one's kidneys were shadowed.

Nick is a musician among the many things he does, and he had one last show out of town very close to the end of our pregnancy. I'd been having flutterings and a few cramps, which I mentioned only under duress since he was so far away. I remained positive, but paid close attention to my body and its signals.

The following weekend, Saturday night, we ended up in the ER. I felt something was off, not quite right. After being admitted, the nurse had me hooked up to the monitors awaiting the doctor on call. My regular doctor was off duty and not returning till Monday morning. Imagine my horror when the new doctor walked in… a member of our gym who I saw regularly! I had no idea he was an ob/gyn. My husband, bless his naiveté, said, "Oh this is great. You'll be ok with him delivering the baby."

Both the doctor and I were shaking our heads, "No." Ladies, you will completely agree with me on this one, won't you?

The concern was, the baby's heart rate kept decelerating when I was lying on my right side. He felt ok with releasing me so long as I promised to call Dr. Chambers first thing Monday and if I would remember to lie on my left side. No way I was forgetting to do that.

Off we went and early Monday I called my ob/gyn. I sent my husband off to work, downtown D.C., with the promise I'd call if there were any issues, but I was feeling ok and baby and I would be fine.

I should have just kept him home! Dr. Chambers sent me back over to the hospital for ultrasounds. By 11am, Nick was back by my side in the hospital because no one was talking to me and starting to upset my zen. More hours, more waiting. And then, around 4pm, Dr. Chambers asked to speak to me. She wanted to induce us that evening. I told her as I'd been telling her, the baby comes out naturally or you can take him out, but you will not be giving me drugs to force it. I have a bad reaction to so many drugs; I was not willing to take the chance.

Thus the c-section was scheduled. Now, in all my research, I'd neglected to really do any reading on c-sections. Why? Probably divine insight. I'm better off not knowing some things, like Lasik surgery… I didn't want to know how they did it, I just wanted to see better. In this case, I just wanted a healthy baby delivered.

Nick darted out to call my mother and her nurse. We'd talked briefly about the fact that I wanted one of the nurses we knew to be in the room with me and for my husband to remain with my mother. One, I didn't really want or need him to see me cut open and two, I really wanted someone there on my side, with a calm head on their shoulders to make sure the doctors and nurses were doing what they're supposed to do!

I remember shivering. I wasn't scared, but the first thing they injected me with made me cold and my muscles just wouldn't stop shivering. Joyce, my nurse, bless her, snapped the ER nurses head off when she commented I was 'just scared'. No, cold. More blankets. Nick went out with my mother and they wheeled me into the surgery room. I still couldn't get the shivers to stop.

Onto the table, the technician with the epidural needed to do his job. "Ma'am, I need to get you to stop shivering so this doesn't hurt you."

I took a deep breath in and just stopped. All muscle movement, all thought, all focus. Everything just stopped.

"How the hell?"

My only response was 'do it quick, I can't hold this forever.'

Epidural was fine, painless, and they got me situated on the table. I was told they would have to strap me down and I said no. They all agreed after the muscle control they'd just seen with the epidural, I'd have no issues.

Twenty-two minutes start to finish. Joyce sat by my head, talking to me the whole time. Dr. Chambers was cheery as ever, fussing at me about how lean I was even with the baby. Then she asked me how I knew? Apparently, our son decided to play jump rope with his umbilical cord, he had it wrapped around his neck and his shoulder. A c-section is the only way he'd have been coming out safely and alive.

His didn't cry at first, calm to start with. I'm not sure what they did, but he wailed suddenly. Finally, they brought him up to lay his cheek next to mine. It is a memory I will never forget.

Then, they were whisking him away, upstairs to check his kidneys. I waited through the stitching, through the family trickling into my room when we were all done… and waited. The grandmothers were wonderful about keeping me sidetracked. Finally the nurse returned with my husband, who was so carefully cradling our son in his arms. Hours after his birth, I was finally able to hold him.

It was an interesting pregnancy. I'd love to do it all over again, but so far, the universe has seen fit to only allow us our son. They grow so fast!

## A Day in the Life of a Midwife: Angel Miller

A typical day in the office in our private practice starts promptly at 0800. Many of the clients I will be seeing today are pregnant, but I am also seeing my recent moms for their annual well woman exams and others for their postpartum exams. It is always a joy to see my moms grow into motherhood and beyond! I am amazed by how our babies grow up before our eyes, as most of my moms bring their babies with them to their visits. I also see a good number of women in their

40's and 50's for their well woman visit too; a nice variety of clients to make the day go by!

My first patient, SR, is complaining of urinary frequency and burning during her well woman visit. After evaluation of her symptoms and a look at her specimen that is sent for culture, I write her a prescription for an antibiotic and bladder analgesic.

A good number of my pregnant clients I am seeing today are term, tired of being pregnant, and just playing the waiting game to give birth to their babies. I discussed Natural Family Planning with AK at her postpartum visit, who would like to have another baby within the year. She is now 9 months postpartum and still breastfeeding. Jacob, her son, is growing by leaps and bounds!

MR had many questions during her well woman exam regarding oral contraception versus the Nuva Ring for her birth control method. She is now 8 months postpartum and is not a good pill taker. She was given a Nuva Ring in the office to try and she loved it! I wrote her a prescription for the next three months to see if she would like to continue with it for the rest of the year.

After seeing clients, reviewing labs, ultrasounds and returning client phone calls, I started my call for the next 24 hours at 7p. After checking with the midwife coming off call, she informed me there was no one in labor. She had one birth earlier in the day and I had two to see for postpartum rounds. Yea! This meant I could go home and have dinner with my family. I had seen several moms that day in the office who were ready to have their babies any day now, so I knew I had to retire early.

At 11pm, my phone rang, and MW called me, a 23 year old primip (first time mom) at 39+ weeks, who told me she thinks she is in labor. Her contractions starting about 1 hour ago. The usual questions were asked of her, how often contractions were, how long they were lasting, any bloody show, any leaking of fluid, is baby moving adequately. She stated her contractions were every seven minutes and lasting 50 seconds. Knowing this was her first baby, I knew I had some wiggle room in getting a few more hours sleep before going in with her. MW was advised to stay hydrated, take a warm shower or bath, and see if the contractions either slow down (false labor) or continue to increase in frequency, intensity and duration. She was talking through her contractions with ease, so I encouraged her also to try and get some rest.

Not 90 minutes later, her husband called and I could hear MW in the background groaning with her contractions and that guttural sound you hear when a woman is in transition. I told her husband that I would meet them at the hospital. Thank God I am only 10 minutes away and the patient was also in close proximity. MW was in labor room #12, and arrived just minutes before I did, and she was fully and ready to push, per the registered nurse!! Not having time to change into scrubs, fashionably in my flip-flops, shorts and t-shirt, I gowned and gloved. I guided MW in her controlled pushing on her left side, and birthed a beautiful baby girl within the next 10 minutes! I am always in awe when moms make it look so easy! "Lily" was put to breast immediately and breastfed like a champ! I was home and in bed within the hour. Knowing I had a long day ahead of me and knowing I was not off the hook by any means, I went right to bed. The birth fairies like to work their magic in the middle of the night.

I was able to sleep until 7a without any interruptions, and went to the hospital to do my postpartum rounds. During that time, I received a call from the midwife in the office who informed me CA, a multip (she was having her fourth baby) at 40 weeks and 1 day, was 5cm dilated and contracting every seven minutes. CA had a history of rapid labors with her 1st and 2nd, so she was strongly encouraged to come to the hospital from the office (a fifteen minute drive). She actually drove herself, parked, and headed to labor and delivery, bags in hand. I met her in the labor room, and she was in a panic because her husband was in D.C. and he was 40 minutes out. She contacted him by phone and that seemed to calm her down, knowing he was on the way. I distracted her with small talk, had her sit on the birthing ball and rubbed her lower back with her contractions. She was progressing nicely and wanted to know how far along she was. I checked her and she was 8cm! (25 minutes after I initially checked her). She again began to panic. "I can't do this on my own! I need an epidural!" I talked to her softly and told her she definitely could do this. She called her husband again to see where he was and he was ten minutes away. This seemed to help her cope and she sat back on the birthing ball, breathing with her contractions and rocking her hips. Her husband came in not five minutes later and CA totally relaxed. It wasn't ten minutes later she had the urge to push, she got on her hands and knees in the bed and pushed twice to crowning, and "Alyssa" was born with a good set of lungs! The baby was passed to CA between her legs, and Alyssa was put to breast immediately, before the placenta was delivered, with CA lying on her side. Both CA and her husband were ecstatic! This was their first girl after three boys.

It was close to 3pm and the labor and delivery floor was buzzing with moms to be. My consulting physician was very busy and had two multips in active labor.

He asked me if I would stand by in Room 9 while he was delivering in Room 7. He stated it was her third baby in Room 9 but hasn't had a baby for nine years. "No problem!" I said. As I was going into Room 9, the nurse had a panicked look on her face. "Her baby is coming now!" I quickly introduced myself, threw on a pair of sterile gloves, no time to gown, and birthed a nine pound four oz. boy with no tears! Baby was placed on Mom's abdomen with a spontaneous cry! Dr. B made it to the room after the placenta was delivered. Both of his patients delivered within two minutes of each other. It goes to show you babies have their own agenda!

Well, believe it or not, this is a typical day in the life of a certified nurse-midwife…

# References

5 Ways to Boost Energy During Pregnancy adapted from www.babyzone.com, Dr. Randy Fink, MD FACOG

American Academy of Pediatrics. 2000. Committee on Substance Abuse and Committee on Children With Disabilities. Policy Statement: Fetal alcohol syndrome and alcohol-related neurodevelopmental disorders. Pediatrics, 106 (2), 358-61.

American College of Obstetricians and Gynecologists (ACOG). 2004. ACOG practice bulletin: Clinical management guidelines for obstetricians-gynecologists. Obstetrics and Gynecology, 103 (4), 803-15.

American Dietetic Association (ADA). 2002. Position of the American Dietetic Association: Nutrition and lifestyle for a healthy pregnancy outcome. Journal of the American Dietetic Association, 102, 1470-90.

Briggs, G. G., Freeman, R. K. and Yaffe, S. *Drugs in Pregnancy and Lactation*, 4th edition. Philadelphia: W. B. Saunders, 1994.

Browne, M.L. 2006. Maternal exposure to caffeine and risk of congenital anomalies: A systematic review. Epidemiology, 17 (3), 324-31.

Centers for Disease Control and Prevention (CDC). 1998. Recommendations to prevent and control iron deficiency in the United States. Morbidity and Mortality Weekly Report (MMWR), 47 (3), 1-36.

Centers for Disease Control and Prevention (CDC). 2005. Use of dietary supplements containing folic acid among women of childbearing age--United States, 2005. MMWR, 54 (38), 955-58.

Clapp, Dr. James F. III, MD. *Exercising Through Your Pregnancy*. Addicus Books: Omaha, Nebraska, 2002. adapted

*Energy in Pregnancy* by Roy M. Pitkin Am J Clin Nutr 1999;69:583. Printed in USA. © 1999 American Society for Clinical Nutrition

Hacker, N., Moore, J.G., & Gambone, J.C. (Eds). 2004. *Essentials of Obstetrics and Gynecology (4th ed.)*. Philadelphia: Saunders.

Henderson, Christine, Jones, Kathleen. *Essentially Midwifery.* "Assessing Maternal and Fetal Well-Being, pages 121-144. Mosby, 1997.

Lewanda, A.F. 2000. *Fetal alcohol syndrome.* Center for Craniofacial Development and Disorders, Johns Hopkins Medical Center.

Mikeska, Erinn, CPT, and Dr. Christine Quatro, *Delivering Fitness.* Brown Books Publishing Group: Dallas, TX, 2004.

Nutrition for you, nutrition for two; "Pregnancy & Lactation" http://www.storknet.com/ip/nutritional_health/basic/pregnancy_guidelines.html

Ritchie, L.D., & King, J.C. 2000. Dietary calcium and pregnancy-induced hypertension: Is there a relation? American Journal of Clinical Nutrition, 71 (5), 1371S-74S.

Riordan, Jan, Auerbach, Kathleen. *Breastfeeding and Human Lactation.* "Anatomy and Psychophysiology of Lactation." Chapter, 4, pages 81-104. Jones and Bartlett Publishers, 1993.

Riordan, Jan, Auerbach, Kathleen. *Breastfeeding and Human Lactation.* "The Breastfeeding Process." Chapter 9, pages 215-247. Jones and Bartlett Publishers, 1993.

Rothman, K.J., et al. 1995. *Teratogenicity of high vitamin A intake.* The New England Journal of Medicine, 333 (21), 1369-73.

Simpkin, P.: Non-pharmacological methods of pain relief during labor. In Chalmers I, Enkin M, Kierse MJNC, editors: *Effective Care in Pregnancy and Childbirth, Vol 2,* Oxford, 1989, Oxford University Press.

U.S. Surgeon General. 2005. News release: U.S. Surgeon General releases advisory on alcohol use in pregnancy, http://www.surgeongeneral.gov/pressreleases/sg02222005.html; retrieved Feb. 4, 2007.

Using illegal street drugs during pregnancy, http://www.americanpregnancy.org/pregnancyhealth/illegaldrugs.html

Varney, Helen, CNM, MSN. *Varney's Midwifery,* Third Edition. "Management Plan for Normal Pregnancy." Pages 249-277. Jones and Bartlett Publishers, 1997.

Womanplace Specialties, Nurse-Midwifery Practice. Common Discomforts in Pregnancy, Wadsworth, Ohio, 2002.

Womanplace Specialties, Nurse-Midwifery Practice. Limiting Weight gain in Pregnancy, Wadsworth, Ohio 2002.

Worthington-Roberts, B, and Rodwell-Williams, S. *Nutrition in Pregnancy and Lactation*, 5th edition: Mosby, 1993. Chapter 11. "Promotion and Support of Breastfeeding." Pages 402-434.


**Additional Resource Websites:**

http://www.babycenter.com/0_calcium-in-your-pregnancy-diet_665.bc#articlesection3

http://my.clevelandclinic.org/health

http://www.mayoclinic.com/health/healthy-baby

http://acnm.org/siteFiles/education/Postpartum_Depression_6_08.pdf

http://www.mymidwife.org/Trimester-by-Trimester

http://www.mymidwife.org/Don-t-Just-Lay-There-Move

http://www.mymidwife.org/Eating-for-Two

http://www.redcrossblood.org/learn-about-blood/health-and-wellness/iron-rich-foods

# About the Authors

**Angel J. Miller, MSN, CNM** is a certified nurse-midwife who has been practicing since 1997. She received her nursing degree in 1986 and her Bachelor of Science and Master of Science Degrees in Nursing at Case Western Reserve University, Cleveland, Ohio. After many years of working as a labor and delivery nurse, Ms. Miller obtained her certification in nurse-midwifery in 1997 by the Frontier School of Midwifery and Family Nursing in Hyden, Kentucky. Ms. Miller continues her strong support for women and women's health and continues to provide excellent midwifery care at Midwifery Care Associates, a nurse midwifery practice located in Rockville, Maryland, just north of the Washington, D.C. area.

**Corry L. Matthews, MS** in Sports Medicine is a fitness and nutrition expert. Her experience includes serving as Gold's Gym International Pre/Postnatal Expert, Elements for Women's Pre/Postnatal Advisory board member, writing for Oxygen (Fit for Two Column) and designing the United States Marine Corps Mom's N Babies Getting Fit Program. Corry lives in Alexandria with her husband, daughter and two dogs.

**Shelia L. Kirkbride, MS** in Rehabilitation Counseling. She has worked in the field of Psychology and Counseling with a wide range of experience in co-occurring psychiatric or emotional illness along with a substance abuse disorders, depression and anxiety, prevention and health, nutrition and weight management, and personal and interpersonal functioning. She is a strong advocate of health and wellness in women's health.

**Stacia D. Kelly, PhD, MHt** is a PhD in Holistic Health, a Master Certified Clinical Hypnotherapist and a Certified Stress Management Specialist. As a martial artist, she teaches her students to achieve balance in body and mind.

# An ACSS Transitions Recommendation

For mothers-to-be and new moms, ACSS Transitions recommends elements™, a premium fitness franchise for **women**, featuring award winning clubs, an acclaimed online magazine, All-Star fitness experts, and so much more!

*Why do we recommend* elements™?

elements™ is a leading fitness and lifestyle brand for women. The company offers fitness and weight loss services through a network of award-winning health clubs, and weight loss centers. In addition, the company features a popular online magazine, media channel (elements living TV), All-Star Fitness Experts and e'co® natural product lines.

elements™ differs from other fitness providers in its "balanced lifestyle" approach to a healthy lifestyle: body, beauty, and mind. The company offers a "total lifestyle" approach to wellness, featuring popular classes and great amenities including smartcard workouts, candlelight yoga, vitality spa™ and more.

## diet and fitness
# elements ™

And as a **Special Offer** to readers of *Nine Months In Nine Months Out…* elements™ invites you to visit any of our locations and receive a FREE two-week pass, just by mentioning this book.

*Make it happen!*™

For locations nearest you, visit elements™ online at
www.elementsforwomen.com.

9 780983 314707